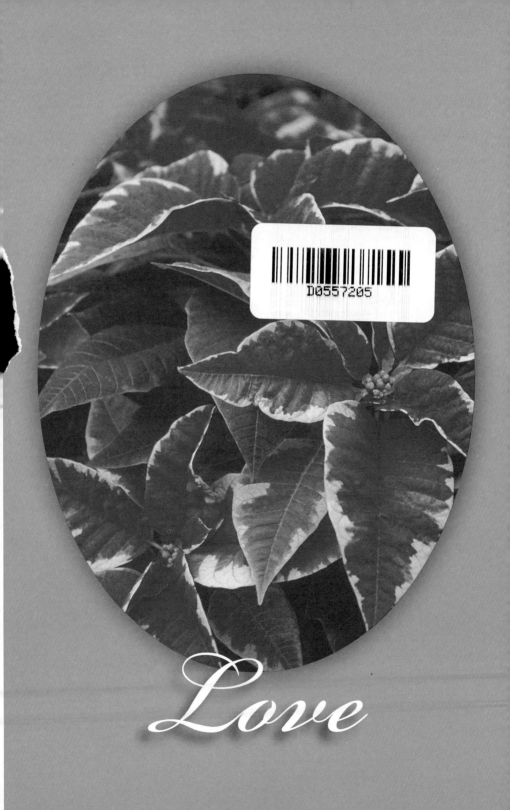

Love

RED DEER LAKE UNITED CHURCH

Calgary, Alberta

www.rdlunitedchurch.org

Advent 4	*Mary Holy Mother*	18 December 2011

Christmas Cantata – Child of Wonder

CALL TO WORSHIP		*Rev. Bob Mutlow*
✞ CAROL	*Gentle Mary Laid Her Child* (Tune: Tempus Adest Floridum)	
LITANY OF MARY		
✞ CAROL	*What Child is this?*	# 74 VU

~Prayer candles may be lit during the singing~

PASSING OF THE PEACE

ANNOUNCEMENTS

✞ ADVENT CANDLE LIGHTING	A *Candle is Burning*	Vs. 1-4 # 6 VU
GOSPEL READING: Luke 1:26-38	*Annunciation*	
MEDITATION	*Mary: Mother in the Faith*	
✞ OFFERTORY	*The Virgin Mary Had a Baby Boy*	# 73 VU

CANATA – Child of Wonder by Lari Goss

Hark the Herald!		
Shine On		
Christmas Makes Me Cry	Soloists	Fran Porter and Juliet Brown
Child of Wonder		
Down in Bethlehem	Dancers: Jenna Den Hoed, Kessa Den Hoed and Hunter Egeland	Trio: Constance Jackson, Kelly Johnson and Juliet Brown
Song to the King	Dancer	Alicia Ward
Heaven is in this House		
Rejoice		
Silent Night! Holy Night!	Children's Chorus	
With Sleep, Baby Jesus	with Adult Choir	
Still the Lamb	Soloist Pat Yerex	
Narrator Andy Porter		
✞ RECESSIONAL	*The First Nowell*	vs. 1-3, 5 & 6 # 91 VU
	The Blessing	

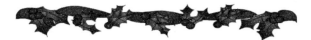

Sopranos
Juliet Brown*
Marj Den Hoed
Marlene Krickhan
Peg Parkin
Fran Porter *
Pat Yerex *

Altos
Pat Claydon
Constance Jackson *
Kelly Johnson *
Colleen Micklethwaite
Thelma Wagner

Basses
Martin Claydon
Roland Eitle
Stan Parkin
Terry Rishaug

Tenors
Doug Den Hoed
John Den Hoed
Greg Ficko

Children's Chorus
John Claydon
Bennet Den Hoed
Britta Den Hoed
Jenna Den Hoed
Kessa Den Hoed
Tara Den Hoed
Hunter Egeland

Children's Chorus
Evia Innes Hayter
Ruth Garana *
Sheila Garana
Hans Vivian
Liesel Vivian

The Sound Team
Rob Claydon
Joe Sherritt

Joseph, Mary and Jesus
Karen, Darren & Baby Ryan Clark

Narrator
Andy Porter

Dancers
Alicia Ward
Jenna Den Hoed,
Kessa Den Hoed and
Hunter Egeland

Drums
Grace Campbell

Children's Choir Director
Cathy Thomsen

Accompanist
Kathy McMullen

Director/ Conductor
Lisa Fernandes

THANK YOU TO OUR VOLUNTEERS

- Voices United Choir Members and CANTATA SINGERS and participants who prepared the Christmas Cantata.
- Greeters: Larry & Gail Stilwell, John & Lois Walker

IN MEMORIUM

- RICHARD SCHELLER (May 06, 1946 – December 09, 2011) spouse of Carol Poffenroth
- CLIFTON STEWART (August 17, 1924 - December 10, 2011) spouse of Lillian Stewart

PRAYER REQUESTS

World Council of Churches Prayer Cycle

- Week 52 – Ghana, Nigeria

Calgary Presbytery United Church of Canada Prayer Cycle

- Ministries & Work of Calgary Presbytery and Lay Delegates

Red Deer Lake United Church Prayer Requests

Contact the Church Office for Prayer Requests to be added to this bulletin.

CHRISTMAS EVE SERVICES @ RDLUC

5:00 – Children's Dress up Pageant for All Ages!

7:00 – Choir Service of Carols & Candles

10:00 – Christmas Eve Communion

Please invite family and friends to join us in a service that fits your family and schedule. All are welcome. There will be no service on Christmas Day. You are invited to join McDougall United Church for a 9:50 "Homespun Christmas Service."

Photo: L. Diane Lackie

The United Church of Canada
L'Église Unie du Canada

MISSION AND
SERVICE FUND

The

Hatha Yoga Pradipika

The
Hatha Yoga Pradipika

The Original Sanskrit
Svatmarama

An English Translation
Brian Dana Akers

YogaVidya.com

An important message to our readers:

The asanas in this book should not be attempted without the supervision of an experienced teacher or prior experience. Many of the other practices should not be attempted at all. The ideas expressed in this book should not be used to diagnose, prescribe, treat, cure, or prevent any disease, illness, or individual health problem. Consult your health care practitioner for individual health care. YogaVidya.com LLC shall not be liable for any direct, indirect, incidental, special, consequential, or punitive damages resulting from the use of this book.

YogaVidya.com, PO Box 569, Woodstock NY 12498-0569 USA

YogaVidya.com and *Read the Originals* are trademarks of YogaVidya.com LLC

First edition

Manufactured in the United States of America

Printed on acid-free paper

Publisher's Cataloging-in-Publication Data

Svatmarama, Swami.
  The Hatha yoga Pradipika / the original Sanskrit [by] Svatmarama ; an English translation [by] Brian Dana Akers.
  Woodstock, NY : YogaVidya.com, 2002.
  xii, [116] p. : ill. ; 23 cm.
  Includes Sanskrit and English.
  ISBN 0-9716466-0-0 (hardcover)
  ISBN 0-9716466-1-9 (paperback)
  1. Yoga, Hatha. 2. Kundalini. I. Title. II. Akers, Brian Dana, 1958-, *tr.*
  BL1238.56.H38   2002
  294.5'436—dc21   2002100228

And would any of this have happened without Loretta?

For Owen & Virginia

Contents

Introduction

Over the last half millennium, one book has established itself as *the* classic work on Hatha Yoga—the book you are holding in your hands. An Indian yogi named Svatmarama wrote the *Hatha Yoga Pradipika* in the fifteenth century C.E. Next to nothing is known about him, although his name may provide a clue. It means "one who delights in one's Atman," indicating the achievement of a state of bliss. Drawing on his own experience and older works now lost, he wrote this book for the student of Yoga. He wrote this book for you.

You've no doubt heard of Hatha Yoga. The word pradipika comes from the Sanskrit verb प्र + दीप् "to flame forth" and means a light, lamp, or lantern. Its extended meaning, since one is throwing light on a subject, is an explanation or commentary. Therefore, the title means "An Explanation of Hatha Yoga."

Even though I've worked hard to make it understandable, this book, like Yoga itself, will require some effort from you. It is chock-full of metaphors, synonyms, and analogies. (Perhaps it also contains a bit of hyperbole.) It is not a smooth, modern narrative, but rather an esoteric work, purposely oblique at times, from medieval India. Furthermore, I recommend that you learn Hatha Yoga under the guidance of an experienced teacher, not solely from this book. Some practices in this book I don't recommend at all.

(You'll know them when you read them.) This is nothing new. Looking at verses 2.37 and 3.22, you can see there have long been different opinions on what should and shouldn't be practiced.

This book is divided into four chapters. In chapter 1, Svatmarama salutes his teachers, says why he is writing this book, who he is writing it for, where and how Yoga should be practiced, describes fifteen asanas, and recommends dietary habits. In chapter 2, he establishes the connections between breath, mind, life, nadis, and prana, then describes the six karmans and the eight kumbhakas. In chapter 3, Svatmarama says what mudras are for, then describes the ten mudras. In chapter 4, he discusses samadhi, laya, nada, two mudras, and the four stages of Yoga.

The Sanskrit original is complete and correct. I carefully examined four previous editions of the text word by word—in fact, letter by letter—to produce the best, most aesthetically pleasing version of the original Sanskrit ever published. I favored more sandhi over less, and took the liberty of simplifying and standardizing the sentence that concludes each chapter. Lines and verses were grouped the way they were translated, but the numbering was left unchanged. I utilized Arabic numerals and left the translation unnumbered to avoid clutter. While including the Sanskrit for the benefit of scholars, students, and posterity, its inclusion—allowing easy comparison with the English—is also a statement of confidence in the quality of the translation.

The English translation is both accurate and accessible. To make it accurate, I stayed in the background and put myself at the service of the author and the text. I suppressed any urges to coin neologisms and employ fleeting usage, or to add my own comments and interpretations. The verse was made the unit of translation to stay off the slippery slope of paraphrase. Where the meaning is open to interpretation, I followed the tradition, specifically Brahmananda's *Jyotsna* commentary. Due to the ever-increasing

knowledge of the reading public, more words were left untrans-
lated than would have been a quarter century ago. (You may want a
dictionary of Yoga handy.) Some previous translators inexplicably
suffocated the book's wonderful parallel constructions; I allowed
them to breathe. The translation is gender neutral where appro-
priate, but many words in the original are gender—even anatomi-
cally—specific, and were left that way. Finally, almost every word
in the original made it into the translation. Few were left out, and
very few new words were added.

I did many things to make the translation accessible. I tried
to use international standard written English and produce prose
that is clear, concise, and direct. To that end, I often broke a long
Sanskrit sentence into shorter English ones, typically changed the
word order from subject-object-verb to subject-verb-object, favored
the active voice over the passive, added the necessary punctuation,
and occasionally moved the latter part of a line or verse to the
beginning for a better flow. Diacritics, italics, and the heavy use of
brackets were dispensed with to avoid the hyperdensity common in
books on Indian philosophy. The transliteration system, therefore,
is not perfect—both श and ष are represented by "sh," for example,
and च is represented by "ch." (However, I retained the familiar Sri
instead of going with Shri, and went with yogi instead of the more
correct yogin.) I invite the stickler for spelling and pronunciation
to learn Devanagari—it's a delightful writing system. Compounds
are generally open to avoid long strings of unfamiliar letter com-
binations, although when compounded, the words bandha, mudra,
kumbhaka, and karman are the final members of a closed compound
for consistency within each category and with the asanas. I decided
notes placed at the foot of the page—rather than at the end of the
chapter, the end of the book, or in brackets within the translation—
would be the least distracting and most convenient way for you to
receive necessary bits of information. Lastly, I regularly changed
the third person potential mood found in many descriptions to a

simple imperative. For example, in verse 1.20, "One should put the right ankle" becomes simply "Put the right ankle."

Knowing a few more things will make this book easier to follow. In Svatmarama's use of language, time equals death, nadis are rivers or streams, chakras are lotuses, sun and moon each refer to multiple things, and the fluid said to drip from a cavity in the skull is variously called soma, nectar, essence, juice, liquor, or crescent water. Kumbhaka means pranayama in general (verse 3.126), breath retention in particular (verse 2.71), and eight specific practices (verse 2.44). Objects means "objects of the senses," and "without objects" more literally means "independent" or "without support." Practices are almost always described before they are named. For example, Simhasana is described in verses 1.50 and 1.51, but not named until verse 1.52. Practices have also changed over the centuries, as have the names attached to them. Indeed, verse 1.37 gives four different names for one asana. In our photographs, we gave primacy to the (often terse and incomplete) descriptions in the book, then filled in the details according to current understanding of the asanas. Appreciation is extended to J. Prabhakara Sastry, who supervised my first attempt at translation in 1979, and to Ashok Aklujkar, who made many last-minute improvements to this effort. Neither is responsible for any remaining shortcomings.

Even keeping all of the above in mind, the meaning of some verses may remain opaque. Rest assured that the translation is complete, clear, and correct. This is an esoteric work from medieval India which describes mystical entities, practices, and states of consciousness. To come to a full realization of Yoga, you will need to study other books, learn from a teacher, and above all, practice.

Finally, you may be wondering if the things described in this book are "really true." I invite the scientifically minded to do some empirical research. In a peaceful country, in a quiet place, free of all anxieties...

प्रथमोपदेशः
Chapter One

Asanas

श्री आदिनाथाय नमोऽस्तु तस्मै येनोपदिष्टा हठयोगविद्या ।
विभ्राजते प्रोन्नतराजयोगमारोढुमिच्छोरधिरोहिणीव ॥ १

Salutations to Shiva, who taught the science of Hatha Yoga.
It is the aspirant's stairway to the heights of Raja Yoga.

प्रणम्य श्रीगुरुं नाथं स्वात्मारामेण योगिना ।
केवलं राजयोगाय हठविद्योपदिश्यते ॥ २

Yogi Svatmarama, after saluting the Lord and guru,
  explains the science of Hatha for one reason—Raja Yoga.

भ्रान्त्या बहुमतध्वान्ते राजयोगमजानताम् ।
हठप्रदीपिकां धत्ते स्वात्मारामः कृपाकरः ॥ ३

For those ignorant of Raja Yoga, wandering in the dark-
ness of too many opinions, compassionate Svatmarama
gives the light of Hatha.

हठविद्यां हि मत्स्येन्द्रगोरक्षाद्या विजानते ।

स्वात्मारामोऽथवा योगी जानीते तत्प्रसादतः ॥ 4

Matsyendra, Goraksha, and others know well the science of Hatha. By their grace, Yogi Svatmarama also knows it.

श्रीआदिनाथमत्स्येन्द्रशाबरानन्दभैरवाः ।
चौरङ्गीमीनगोरक्षविरूपाक्षबिलेशयाः ॥ 5
मन्थानो भैरवो योगी सिद्धिर्बुद्धश्च कन्थडिः ।
कोरण्टकः सुरानन्दः सिद्धपादश्च चर्पटिः ॥ 6
कानेरी पूज्यपादश्च नित्यनाथो निरञ्जनः ।
कपाली बिन्दुनाथश्च काकचण्डीश्वराह्वयः ॥ 7
अल्लामः प्रभुदेवश्च घोडाचोली च टिण्टिणिः ।
भानुकी नारदेवश्च खण्डः कापालिकस्तथा ॥ 8
इत्यादयो महासिद्धा हठयोगप्रभावतः ।
खण्डयित्वा कालदण्डं ब्रह्माण्डे विचरन्ति ते ॥ 9

Shiva, Matsyendra, Shabara, Anandabhairava, Chaurangi, Mina, Goraksha, Virupaksha, Bileshaya, Manthana, Bhairava, Siddhi, Buddha, Kanthadi, Korantaka, Surananda, Siddhapada, Charpati, Kaneri, Pujyapada, Nityanatha, Niranjana, Kapali, Bindunatha, Kakachandishvara, Allama Prabhudeva, Ghodacholi, Tintini, Bhanuki, Naradeva, Khanda, and Kapalika—these and other great masters, having conquered death through the power of Hatha Yoga, roam the universe.

अशेषतापतप्तानां समाश्रयमठो हठः ।

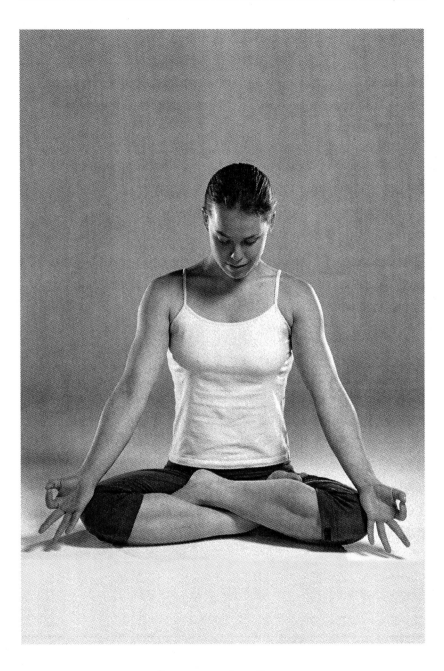

स्वस्तिकासन – Svastikasana

अशेषयोगयुक्तानामाधारकमठो हठः ॥ 10

Hatha is the sanctuary for those suffering every type of pain. It is the foundation for those practicing every type of Yoga.

हठविद्या परं गोप्या योगिना सिद्धिमिच्छता ।
भवेद्वीर्यवती गुप्ता निर्वीर्या तु प्रकाशिता ॥ 11

The science of Hatha should be kept top secret by the yogi desirous of success. It is potent when concealed and impotent when revealed.

सुराज्ये धार्मिके देशे सुभिक्षे निरुपद्रवे ।
धनुःप्रमाणपर्यन्ते शिलाग्निजलवर्जिते ।
एकान्ते मठिकामध्ये स्थातव्यं हठयोगिना ॥ 12

The Hatha yogi should live in a secluded hut free of stones, fire, and dampness to a distance of four cubits in a country that is properly governed, virtuous, prosperous, and peaceful.

अल्पद्वारमरन्ध्रगर्तविवरं नात्युच्चनीचायतं
सम्यग्गोमयसान्द्रलिप्तममलं निःशेषजन्तूज्झितम् ।
बाह्ये मण्डपवेदिकूपरुचिरं प्राकारसंवेष्टितं
प्रोक्तं योगमठस्य लक्षणमिदं सिद्धैर्हठाभ्यासिभिः ॥ 13

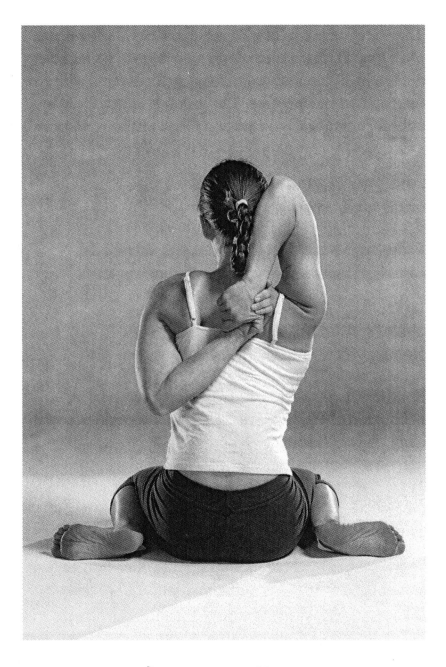

गोमुखासन – Gomukhasana

These are the marks of a Yoga hut as described by masters practicing Hatha: a small door, no windows, no rat holes; not too high, too low, or too long; well plastered with cow dung, clean, and bug free. The grounds are enclosed by a wall and beautified by an arbor, a raised platform, and a well.

एवंविधे मठे स्थित्वा सर्वचिन्ताविवर्जितः ।
गुरूपदिष्टमार्गेण योगमेव समभ्यसेत् ॥ 14

Living in this hut, free of all anxieties, one should earnestly practice Yoga as taught by one's guru.

अत्याहारः प्रयासश्च प्रजल्पो नियमग्रहः ।
जनसङ्गश्च लौल्यं च षड्भिर्योगो विनश्यति ॥ 15

Yoga perishes by these six: overeating, overexertion, talking too much, performing needless austerities, socializing, and restlessness.

उत्साहात्साहसाद्धैर्यात्तत्त्वज्ञानाच्च निश्चयात् ।
जनसङ्गपरित्यागात्षड्भिर्योगः प्रसिद्ध्यति ॥ 16

Yoga succeeds by these six: enthusiasm, openness, courage, knowledge of the truth, determination, and solitude.

हठस्य प्रथमाङ्गत्वादासनं पूर्वमुच्यते ।
कुर्यात्तदासनं स्थैर्यमारोग्यं चाङ्गलाघवम् ॥ 17

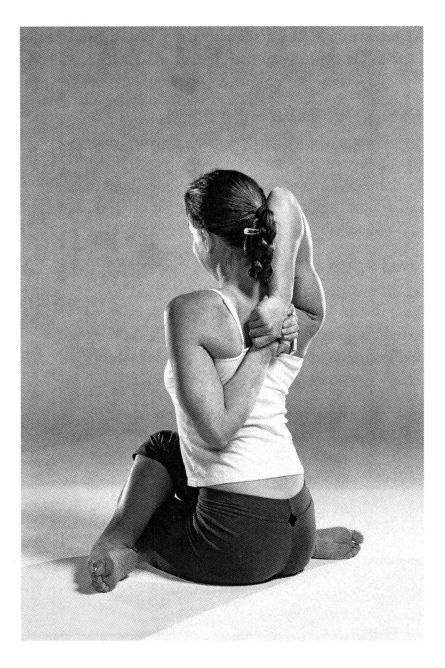

वीरासन – Virasana

Asanas are described first because they are the first step of Hatha. They give steadiness, health, and lightness of body.

वसिष्ठाद्यैश्च मुनिभिर्मत्स्येन्द्राद्यैश्च योगिभिः ।
अङ्गीकृतान्यासनानि कथ्यन्ते कानिचिन्मया ॥ 18

I will describe some asanas endorsed by Vasishtha and other sages, and by Matsyendra and other yogis.

जानूर्वोरन्तरे सम्यक्कृत्वा पादतले उभे ।
ऋजुकायः समासीनः स्वस्तिकं तत्प्रचक्षते ॥ 19

Correctly place both soles of the feet inside the thighs and knees. Sit up straight. This is Svastikasana.

सव्ये दक्षिणगुल्फं तु पृष्ठपार्श्वे नियोजयेत् ।
दक्षिणेऽपि तथा सव्यं गोमुखं गोमुखाकृति ॥ 20

Put the right ankle on its left side beside the buttock. Likewise, put the left ankle on its right side. This is called Gomukhasana because it resembles a cow's face.

एकं पादं तथैकस्मिन्विन्यसेदूरुणि स्थितम् ।
इतरस्मिंस्तथा चोरुं वीरासनमितीरितम् ॥ 21

Similarly, place one foot on top of one thigh, and the other thigh on top of the other foot. This is Virasana.

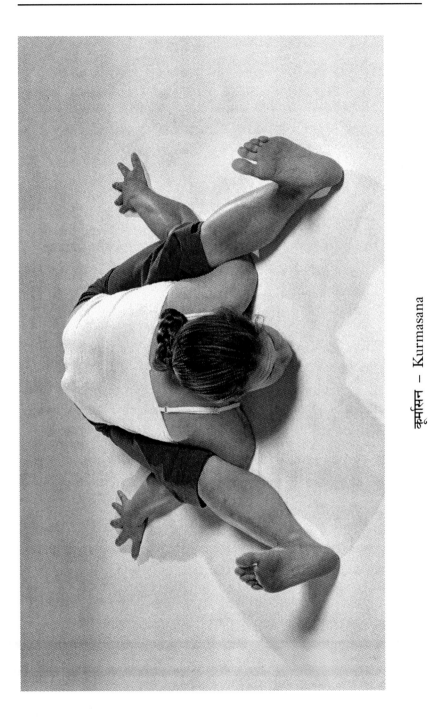

कूर्मासन – Kurmasana

गुदं निरुध्य गुल्फाभ्यां व्युत्क्रमेण समाहितः ।
कूर्मासनं भवेदेतदिति योगविदो विदुः ॥ 22

Cover the anus with crossed ankles and sit motionless.
Knowers of Yoga know that this is Kurmasana.[1]

पद्मासनं तु संस्थाप्य जानूर्वोरन्तरे करौ ।
निवेश्य भूमौ संस्थाप्य व्योमस्थं कुक्कुटासनम् ॥ 23

Settle in Padmasana. Put the hands between the knees
and thighs. Place the hands on the earth. Lift into the sky.
This is Kukkutasana.

कुक्कुटासनबन्धस्थो दोर्भ्यां संबध्य कन्धराम् ।
भवेत्कूर्मवदुत्तान एतदुत्तानकूर्मकम् ॥ 24

Assume Kukkutasana, join the neck with the hands, and
lie on the back like a turtle. This is Uttanakurmasana.

पादाङ्गुष्ठौ तु पाणिभ्यां गृहीत्वा श्रवणावधि ।
धनुराकर्षणं कुर्याद्धनुरासनमुच्यते ॥ 25

Bring the big toes as far as the ears with both hands as if
drawing a bow. This is Dhanurasana.

वामोरुमूलार्पितदक्षपादं जानोर्बहिर्वेष्टितवामपादम् ।

---

[1] The asana nowadays called Kurmasana no longer corresponds to this
description. We have photographed the modern version.

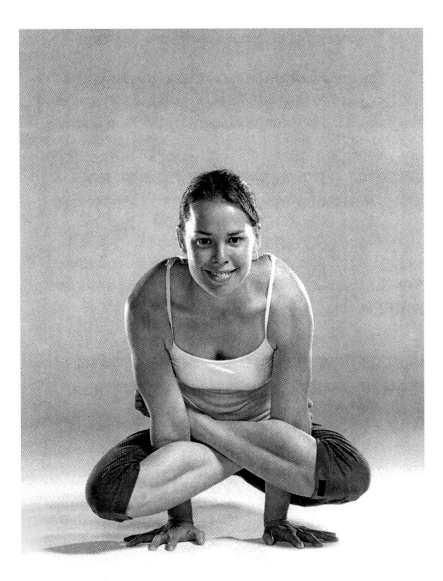

कुक्कुटासन – Kukkutasana

प्रगृह्य तिष्ठेत्परिवर्तिताङ्गः श्रीमत्स्यनाथोदितमासनं स्यात् ॥ 26

Place the right foot at the root of the left thigh, and the left foot outside the right knee. Grasp the feet and twist the body. This is the asana taught by Sri Matsyanatha.

मत्स्येन्द्रपीठं जठरप्रदीप्तिं प्रचण्डरुग्मण्डलखण्डनास्त्रम् ।
अभ्यासतः कुण्डलिनीप्रबोधं चन्द्रस्थिरत्वं च ददाति पुंसाम् ॥ 27

This Matsyendrasana stimulates the appetite. It is a weapon which destroys a multitude of deadly diseases. Regular practice awakens the kundalini and firms the moon[2] in men.

प्रसार्य पादौ भुवि दण्डरूपौ दोर्भ्यां पदाग्रद्वितयं गृहीत्वा ।
जानूपरि न्यस्तललाटदेशो वसेदिदं पश्चिमतानमाहुः ॥ 28

Stretch both legs on the ground like sticks. Grasp the toes with both hands. Rest the forehead on the knees. This is Paschimatanasana.

इति पश्चिमतानमासनाग्र्यं पवनं पश्चिमवाहिनं करोति ।
उदयं जठरानलस्य कुर्यादुदरे काश्यर्यमरोगतां च पुंसाम् ॥ 29

This Paschimatana is foremost among asanas. It reverses the breath's flow, kindles the fire of the stomach, flattens the belly, and brings good health to men.

---

[2] Discussion of this meaning of the word moon begins with verse 3.49.

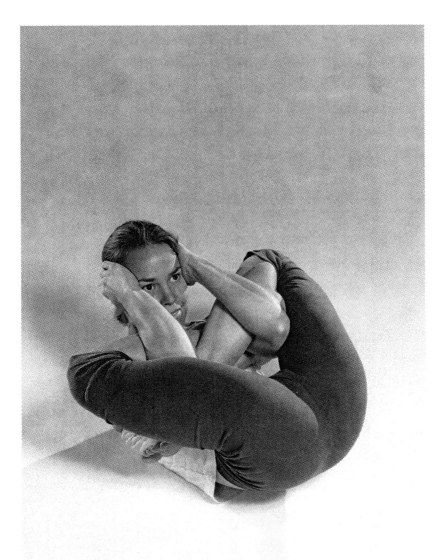

उत्तानकूर्मासन – Uttanakurmasana

धरामवष्टभ्य करद्वयेन तत्कूर्परस्थापितनाभिपार्श्वः ।
उच्चासनो दण्डवदुत्थितः स्यान्मायूरमेतत्प्रवदन्ति पीठम् ॥ 30

Hold the earth with both hands. Place the sides of the
navel on the elbows. Rise high above the ground like a
stick. This is Mayurasana.

हरति सकलरोगानाशु गुल्मोदरादी-
नभिभवति च दोषानासनं श्रीमयूरम् ।
बहु कदशनभुक्तं भस्म कुर्यादशेषं
जनयति जठराग्निं जारयेत्कालकूटम् ॥ 31

The Sri Mayurasana overcomes defects and quickly
destroys all diseases—enlargement of the spleen, enlargement of the abdomen, and so on. It stimulates the
stomach's fire, incinerates all bad food, and makes the
deadly Kalakuta poison digestible.

उत्तानं शववद्भूमौ शयनं तच्छवासनम् ।
शवासनं श्रान्तिहरं चित्तविश्रान्तिकारकम् ॥ 32

Lying on the back on the ground like a corpse is
Shavasana. It removes fatigue and gives rest to the mind.

चतुरशीत्यासनानि शिवेन कथितानि च ।
तेभ्यश्चतुष्कमादाय सारभूतं ब्रवीम्यहम् ॥ 33

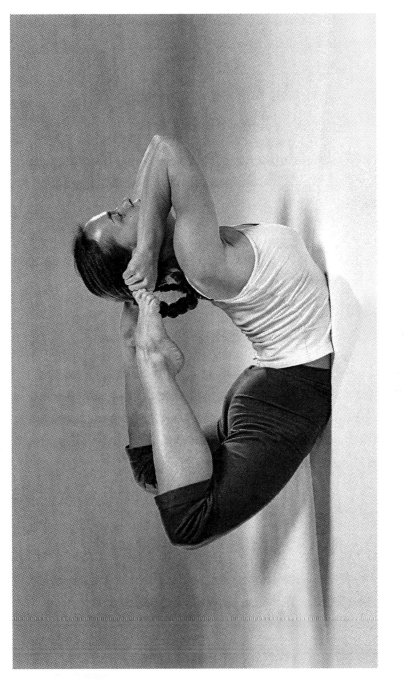

धनुरासन – Dhanurasana

Eighty-four asanas were taught by Shiva. Of those I shall describe the essential four.

सिद्धं पद्मं तथा सिंहं भद्रं चेति चतुष्टयम् ।
श्रेष्ठं तत्रापि च सुखे तिष्ठेत्सिद्धासने सदा ॥ 34

Siddha, Padma, Simha, and Bhadra—these four are the best. And of these, Siddhasana is always comfortable to maintain.

योनिस्थानकमङ्घ्रिमूलघटितं कृत्वा दृढं विन्यसे-
न्मेण्ढ्रे पादमथैकमेव हृदये कृत्वा हनुं सुस्थिरम् ।
स्थाणुः संयमितेन्द्रियोऽचलदृशा पश्येद्भुवोरन्तरं
होतन्मोक्षकपाटभेदजनकं सिद्धासनं प्रोच्यते ॥ 35

Press the perineum with the heel of the foot. Place the other foot above the penis. Hold the chin steady on the heart. Remain motionless. Restrain the senses. Look with a steady gaze between the eyebrows. This is Siddhasana. It opens the doors of liberation.

मेण्ढ्रादुपरि विन्यस्य सव्यं गुल्फं तथोपरि ।
गुल्फान्तरं च निक्षिप्य सिद्धासनमिदं भवेत् ॥ 36

Place the left ankle above the penis. Put the other ankle above the left foot. Some say this is Siddhasana.

एतत्सिद्धासनं प्राहुरन्ये वज्रासनं विदुः ।

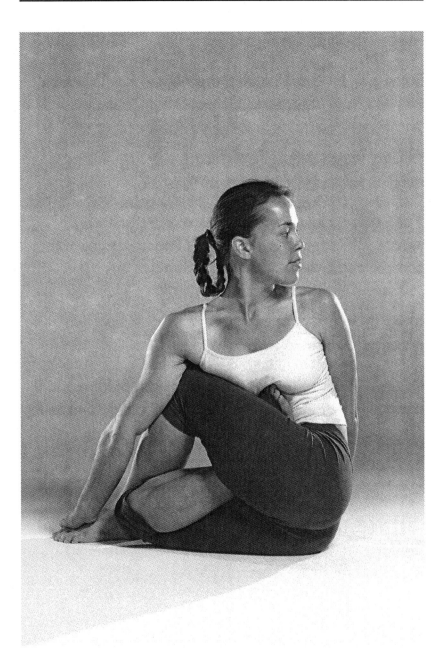

मत्स्येन्द्रासन – Matsyendrasana

मुक्तासनं वदन्त्येके प्राहुर्गुप्तासनं परे ॥ 37

Some call this Siddhasana. Others know it as Vajrasana. Some say it is Muktasana. Others call it Guptasana.

यमेष्विव मिताहारमहिंसां नियमेष्विव ।
मुख्यं सर्वासनेष्वेकं सिद्धाः सिद्धासनं विदुः ॥ 38

The masters know that Siddhasana is the best of all asanas, just as moderate diet is the foremost yama and nonviolence is the fundamental niyama.

चतुरशीतिपीठेषु सिद्धमेव सदाभ्यसेत् ।
द्वासप्ततिसहस्राणां नाडीनां मलशोधनम् ॥ 39

Of the eighty-four asanas, always practice Siddhasana. It removes impurities from the seventy-two thousand nadis.

आत्मध्यायी मिताहारी यावद्द्वादशवत्सरम् ।
सदा सिद्धासनाभ्यासाद्योगी निष्पत्तिमाप्नुयात् ॥ 40

The yogi will obtain fulfillment through self-contemplation, eating moderately, and practicing Siddhasana regularly for twelve years.

किमन्यैर्बहुभिः पीठैः सिद्धे सिद्धासने सति ।
प्राणानिले सावधाने बद्धे केवलकुम्भके ।
उत्पद्यते निरायासात्स्वयमेवोन्मनी कला ॥ 41

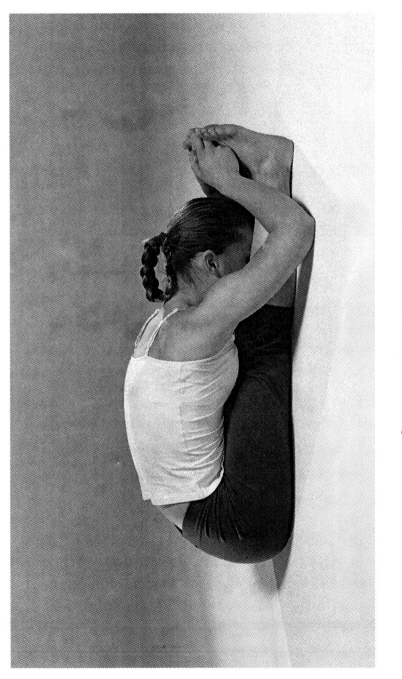

पश्चिमतानासन – Paschimatanasana

What use are the many other asanas once Siddhasana is perfected? When the prana is restrained with concentration in Kevalakumbhaka, the unmani pleasure arises easily by itself.

तथैकस्मिन्नेव दृढे सिद्धे सिद्धासने सति ।
बन्धत्रयमनायासात्स्वयमेवोपजायते ॥ 42

When the one and only Siddhasana is solid and perfected, the three bandhas[3] arise easily by themselves.

नासनं सिद्धसदृशं न कुम्भः केवलोपमः ।
न खेचरीसमा मुद्रा न नादसदृशो लयः ॥ 43

There is no asana like Siddha, no kumbhaka comparable to Kevala, no mudra equal to Khechari, no laya like nada.

वामोरूपरि दक्षिणं च चरणं संस्थाप्य वामं तथा
दक्षोरूपरि पश्चिमेन विधिना धृत्वा कराभ्यां दृढम् ।
अङ्गुष्ठौ हृदये निधाय चिबुकं नासाग्रमालोकये-
देतद्व्याधिविनाशकारि यमिनां पद्मासनं प्रोच्यते ॥ 44

Place the right foot above the left thigh and the left foot above the right thigh. Hold the big toes firmly with both hands brought from behind. Put the chin on the heart. Look at the tip of the nose. This is Padmasana. It destroys the sickness of those who practice it.

---

[3] Jalandharabandha, Uddiyanabandha, and Mulabandha.

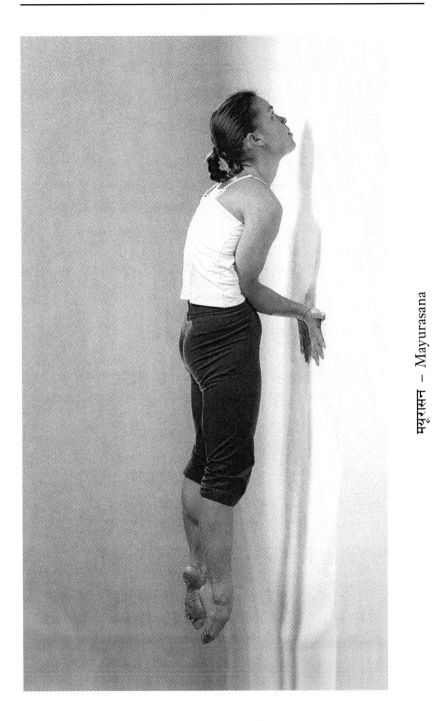

मयूरासन – *Mayurasana*

उत्तानौ चरणौ कृत्वा ऊरुसंस्थौ प्रयत्नतः ।
ऊरुमध्ये तथोत्तानौ पाणी कृत्वा ततो दृशौ ॥ 45
नासाग्रे विन्यसेद्राजदन्तमूले तु जिह्वया ।
उत्तम्भ्य चिबुकं वक्षस्युत्थाप्य पवनं शनैः ॥ 46

Drag the upturned feet onto the thighs. Place the upturned hands in the middle of the thighs. Keep the eyes on the tip of the nose. Hold the root of the front teeth with the tongue. Place the chin on the chest. Slowly lift the wind upward.

इदं पद्मासनं प्रोक्तं सर्वव्याधिविनाशनम् ।
दुर्लभं येन केनापि धीमता लभ्यते भुवि ॥ 47

Some call this Padmasana. It is the destroyer of all diseases. Not just anyone can have it. Only the wise on earth attain it.

कृत्वा संपुटितौ करौ दृढतरं बद्ध्वा तु पद्मासनं
गाढं वक्षसि संनिधाय चिबुकं ध्यायंश्च तच्चेतसि ।
वारं वारमपानमूर्ध्वमनिलं प्रोत्सारयन्पूरितं
न्यञ्जन्प्राणमुपैति बोधमतुलं शक्तिप्रभावान्नरः ॥ 48

Form a solid Padmasana. Clasp the hands together. Put the chin firmly on the chest. Contemplate the Absolute in the mind. Repeatedly move the apana wind upwards and the inhaled prana downwards. Thus a man reaches unequaled knowledge from the power of shakti.

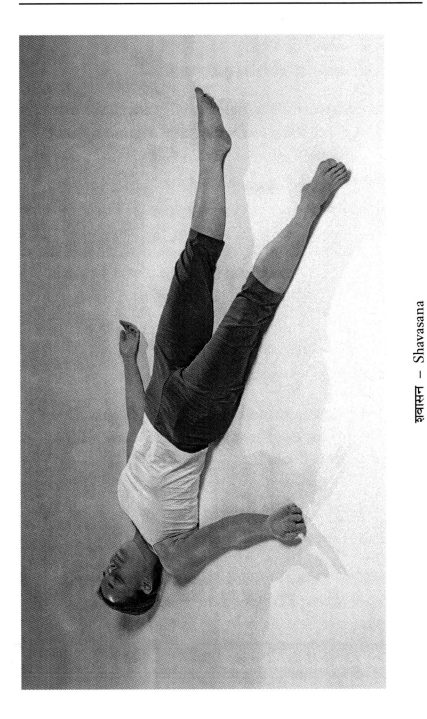

शवासन – Shavasana

पद्मासने स्थितो योगी नाडीद्वारेण पूरितम् ।
मारुतं धारयेद्यस्तु स मुक्तो नात्र संशयः ॥ 49

The yogi who sits in Padmasana and holds the breath
inhaled through the nadis is liberated without a doubt.

गुल्फौ च वृषणस्याधः सीवन्याः पार्श्वयोः क्षिपेत् ।
दक्षिणे सव्यगुल्फं तु दक्षगुल्फं तु सव्यके ॥ 50

Place the ankles below the scrotum on both sides of the
perineum—the left ankle on the right, the right ankle
on the left.

हस्तौ तु जान्वोः संस्थाप्य स्वाङ्गुलीः संप्रसार्य च ।
व्यात्तवक्त्रो निरीक्षेत नासाग्रं सुसमाहितः ॥ 51

Place the hands on the knees. Spread the fingers. Open
the mouth. Gaze steadily at the tip of the nose with a
well-concentrated mind.

सिंहासनं भवेदेतत्पूजितं योगिपुङ्गवैः ।
बन्धत्रितयसंधानं कुरुते चासनोत्तमम् ॥ 52

This is Simhasana. It is honored by the best of yogis.
This supreme asana connects the three bandhas.

गुल्फौ च वृषणस्याधः सीवन्याः पार्श्वयोः क्षिपेत् ।
सव्यगुल्फं तथा सव्ये दक्षगुल्फं तु दक्षिणे ॥ 53

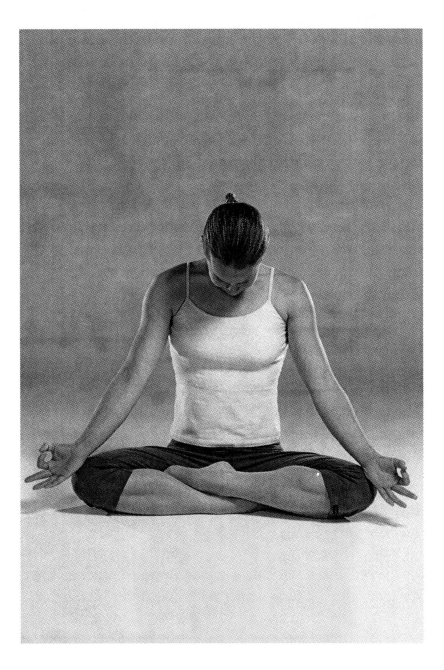

सिद्धासन – Siddhasana

Place the ankles below the scrotum on both sides of the
perineum—the left ankle on the left, the right ankle
on the right.

पार्श्वपादौ च पाणिभ्यां दृढं बद्ध्वा सुनिश्चलम् ।
भद्रासनं भवेदेतत्सर्वव्याधिविनाशनम् ।
गोरक्षासनमित्याहुरिदं वै सिद्धयोगिनः ॥ 54

Grasp the feet, which are on their sides, firmly with
the hands. Remain motionless. This is Bhadrasana. It
is the destroyer of all diseases. Expert yogis call this
Gorakshasana.

एवमासनबन्धेषु योगीन्द्रो विगतश्रमः ।
अभ्यसेन्नाडिकाशुद्धिं मुद्रादिपवनक्रियाम् ॥ 55

The best yogis, holding asanas and bandhas without
fatigue, should purify the nadis with pranayama, mudras,
and so on.

आसनं कुम्भकं चित्रं मुद्राख्यं करणं तथा ।
अथ नादानुसंधानमभ्यासानुक्रमो हठे ॥ 56

Asanas, various kumbhakas, practices called mudras, then
concentration on nada—this is Hatha's order of practice.

ब्रह्मचारी मिताहारी त्यागी योगपरायणः ।
अब्दादूर्ध्वं भवेत्सिद्धो नात्र कार्या विचारणा ॥ 57

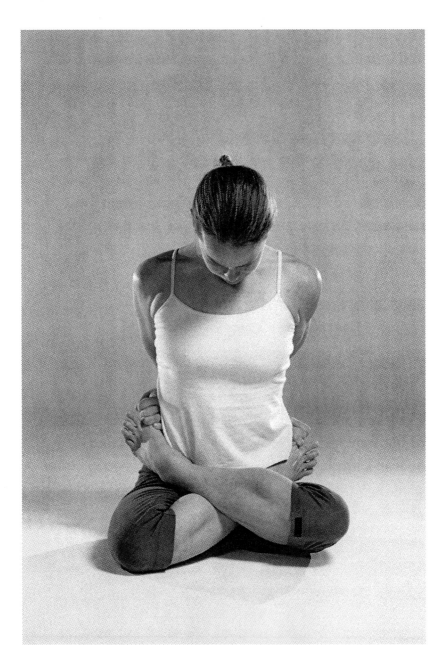

पद्मासन – Padmasana

One who is a brahmachari, a moderate eater, a renouncer, and intent on Yoga will be an expert after a year. In this there is no doubt.

सुस्निग्धमधुराहारश्चतुर्थांशविवर्जितः ।
भुज्यते शिवसंप्रीत्यै मिताहारः स उच्यते ॥ 58

A moderate diet means eating satisfying, sweet food for Shiva's pleasure, while leaving the stomach one-quarter empty.

कट्वम्लतीक्ष्णलवणोष्णहरीतशाक-
सौवीरतैलतिलसर्षपमद्यमत्स्यान् ।
आजादिमांसदधितक्रकुलत्थकोल-
पिण्याकहिङ्गुलशुनाद्यमपथ्यमाहुः ॥ 59

These are not recommended: bitter, sour, spicy, salty, or hot food; green leaves, sour gruel, oil, sesame seeds, mustard, alcohol, fish, goat or other meat, curds, butter-milk, kulattha pulses, kola berries, oil cake, asafetida, garlic, and so on.

भोजनमहितं विद्यात्पुनरस्योष्णीकृतं रूक्षम् ।
अतिलवणमम्लयुक्तं कद्शनशाकोत्कटं वर्ज्यम् ॥ 60

Food that is reheated, parched, too salty, too sour, or contains too many stale vegetables is improper and should be avoided.

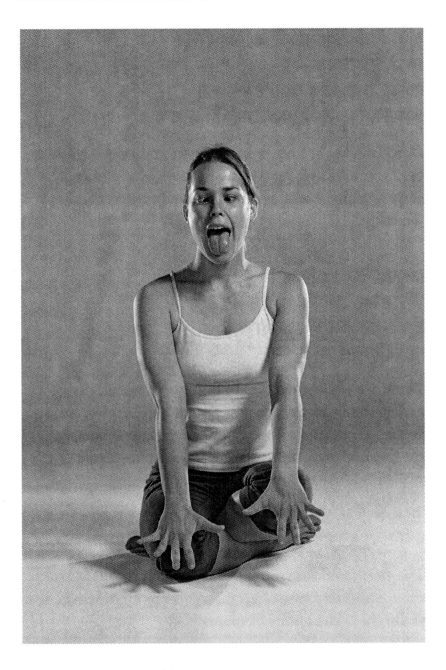

सिंहासन – Simhasana

वह्निस्त्रीपथिसेवानामादौ वर्जनमाचरेत् ।
तथाहि गोरक्षवचनम् ।
वर्जयेद्दुर्जनप्रान्तं वह्निस्त्रीपथिसेवनम् ।
प्रातःस्नानोपवासादि कायक्लेशविधिं तथा ॥ 61

Don't indulge in fires, women, or travel in the beginning.
For Goraksha says: Avoid bad people, fires, women, travel,
early morning baths, fasting, etc., and actions that hurt
the body.

गोधूमशालियवषाष्टिकशोभनान्नं
क्षीराज्यखण्डनवनीतसितामधूनि ।
शुण्ठीपटोलकफलादिकपञ्चशाकं
मुद्गादिदिव्यमुदकं च यमीन्द्रपथ्यम् ॥ 62

These are wholesome for the best yogis: wheat, rice,
barley, shashtika rice, auspicious food, milk, ghee, sugar,
butter, sugar candy, honey, dry ginger, cucumbers, etc.,
the five potherbs, mung dahl, etc., and pure water.

पुष्टं सुमधुरं स्निग्धं गव्यं धातुप्रपोषणम् ।
मनोभिलषितं योग्यं योगी भोजनमाचरेत् ॥ 63

The yogi should eat food that is desirable, suitable, nutri-
tious, pleasantly sweet, juicy, contains dairy products, and
strengthens the bodily elements.

युवा वृद्धोऽतिवृद्धो वा व्याधितो दुर्बलोऽपि वा ।

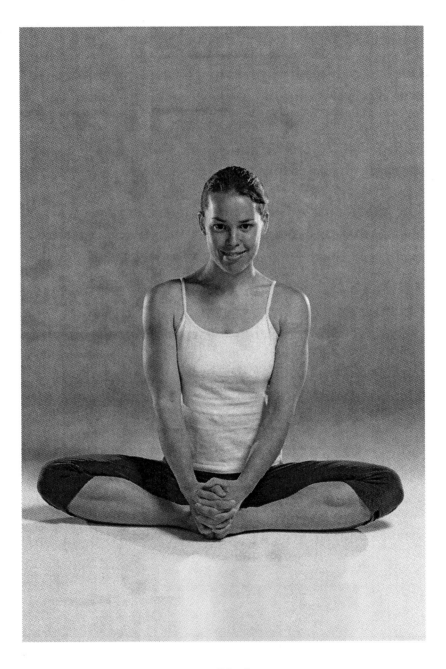

भद्रासन – Bhadrasana

अभ्यासात्सिद्धिमाप्नोति सर्वयोगेष्वतन्द्रितः ॥ 64

One succeeds in all Yogas through energetic practice—
even if one is young, old, very old, sick, or weak.

क्रियायुक्तस्य सिद्धिः स्यादक्रियस्य कथं भवेत् ।
न शास्त्रपाठमात्रेण योगसिद्धिः प्रजायते ॥ 65

The practitioner will succeed; the nonpractitioner will not.
Success in Yoga is not achieved by merely reading books.

न वेषधारणं सिद्धेः कारणं न च तत्कथा ।
क्रियैव कारणं सिद्धेः सत्यमेतन्न संशयः ॥ 66

Success is achieved neither by wearing the right clothes
nor by talking about it. Practice alone brings success.
This is the truth, without a doubt.

पीठानि कुम्भकाश्चित्रा दिव्यानि करणानि च ।
सर्वाण्यपि हठाभ्यासे राजयोगफलावधि ॥ 67

Practice Hatha's asanas, various kumbhakas, and excellent
karanas until the fruit of Raja Yoga is won.

इति हठयोगप्रदीपिकायां प्रथमोपदेशः ॥

Thus ends the first chapter in the Hatha Yoga Pradipika.

द्वितीयोपदेशः

Chapter Two

Pranayama

अथासने दृढे योगी वशी हितमिताशनः ।
गुरूपदिष्टमार्गेण प्राणायामान्समभ्यसेत् ॥ 1

After mastering asanas, the yogi—possessing self-control and eating a suitable, moderate diet—should practice pranayama as taught by his guru.

चले वाते चलं चित्तं निश्चले निश्चलं भवेत् ।
योगी स्थाणुत्वमाप्नोति ततो वायुं निरोधयेत् ॥ 2

When the breath is unsteady, the mind is unsteady. When the breath is steady, the mind is steady, and the yogi becomes steady. Therefore one should restrain the breath.

यावद्वायुः स्थितो देहे तावज्जीवनमुच्यते ।
मरणं तस्य निष्क्रान्तिस्ततो वायुं निरोधयेत् ॥ 3

As long as there is breath in the body, there is life. Death is the departure of breath. Therefore one should restrain the breath.

मलाकुलासु नाडीषु मारुतो नैव मध्यगः ।
कथं स्यादुन्मनीभावः कार्यसिद्धिः कथं भवेत् ॥ 4

When the nadis are disrupted by impurities, the breath doesn't enter the middle.[1] How can unmani exist? How can the goal be attained?

शुद्धिमेति यदा सर्वं नाडीचक्रं मलाकुलम् ।
तदैव जायते योगी प्राणसंग्रहणे क्षमः ॥ 5

The yogi is fit to control the prana only when all the nadis disrupted by impurities become pure.

प्राणायामं ततः कुर्यान्नित्यं सात्त्विकया धिया ।
यथा सुषुम्नानाडीस्था मलाः शुद्धिं प्रयान्ति च ॥ 6

Therefore always do pranayama with a sattvik mind so that impurities in the Sushumna nadi attain purity.

बद्धपद्मासनो योगी प्राणं चन्द्रेण पूरयेत् ।
धारयित्वा यथाशक्ति भूयः सूर्येण रेचयेत् ॥ 7

The yogi, having assumed Padmasana, should inhale prana with the moon.[2] After holding as long as possible, he should exhale with the sun.[3]

---

[1] The Sushumna.
[2] The left nostril, or Ida.
[3] The right nostril, or Pingala.

प्राणं सूर्येण चाकृष्य पूरयेदुदरं शनैः ।
विधिवत्कुम्भकं कृत्वा पुनश्चन्द्रेण रेचयेत् ॥ 8

He should fill the interior slowly by inhaling prana with
the sun. After holding in the prescribed manner, he
should exhale with the moon.

येन त्यजेत्तेन पीत्वा धारयेदतिरोधतः ।
रेचयेञ्च ततोऽन्येन शनैरेव न वेगतः ॥ 9

He should inhale through the one with which he exhaled,
hold with effort, then exhale slowly and without force
through the other.

प्राणं चेदिडया पिबेन्नियमितं भूयोऽन्यया रेचयेत्
पीत्वा पिङ्गलया समीरणमथो बद्ध्वा त्यजेद्वामया ।
सूर्याचन्द्रमसोरनेन विधिनाभ्यासं सदा तन्वतां
शुद्धा नाडिगणा भवन्ति यमिनां मासत्रयादूर्ध्वतः ॥ 10

If prana is inhaled through the Ida and retained, it should
be exhaled through the other. If the breath is inhaled
through the Pingala and retained, it should be exhaled
through the left. The nadis of yogis who regularly
practice in this manner of sun and moon become pure
after three months.

प्रातर्मध्यन्दिने सायमर्धरात्रे च कुम्भकान् ।
शनैरशीतिपर्यन्तं चतुर्वारं समभ्यसेत् ॥ 11

Gradually increase the kumbhakas to eighty, four times a day—morning, midday, evening, and midnight.

कनीयसि भवेत्स्वेदः कम्पो भवति मध्यमे ।
उत्तमे स्थानमाप्नोति ततो वायुं निबन्धयेत् ॥ 12

In the beginning there will be sweat. In the middle there is trembling. In the end, one obtains the goal. Therefore one should restrain the breath.

जलेन श्रमजातेन गात्रमर्दनमाचरेत् ।
दृढता लघुता चैव तेन गात्रस्य जायते ॥ 13

Rub the body with the water born of fatigue to make it firm and light.

अभ्यासकाले प्रथमे शस्तं क्षीराज्यभोजनम् ।
ततोऽभ्यासे दृढीभूते न तादृङ्नियमग्रहः ॥ 14

Food containing milk and ghee is recommended for the initial phase of practice. The adoption of such a rule is unnecessary after one's practice is established.

यथा सिंहो गजो व्याघ्रो भवेद्वश्यः शनैः शनैः ।
तथैव सेवितो वायुरन्यथा हन्ति साधकम् ॥ 15

Just as a lion, elephant, or tiger is tamed step by step, so the breath is controlled. Otherwise it kills the practitioner.

प्राणायामेन युक्तेन सर्वरोगक्षयो भवेत् ।
अयुक्ताभ्यासयोगेन सर्वरोगसमुद्भवः ॥ 16

Correct pranayama will weaken all diseases. Improper
practice of Yoga will strengthen all diseases.

हिक्का श्वासश्च कासश्च शिरःकर्णाक्षिवेदनाः ।
भवन्ति विविधा रोगाः पवनस्य प्रकोपतः ॥ 17

Irritation of the breath causes hiccups, asthma, coughing,
headaches, earaches, pain in the eyes, and various diseases.

युक्तं युक्तं त्यजेद्वायुं युक्तं युक्तं च पूरयेत् ।
युक्तं युक्तं च बध्नीयादेवं सिद्धिमवाप्नुयात् ॥ 18

Exhale the breath very properly. Inhale it very properly.
Retain it very properly. Thus one obtains success.

यदा तु नाडीशुद्धिः स्यात्तथा चिह्नानि बाह्यतः ।
कायस्य कृशता कान्तिस्तदा जायेत निश्चितम् ॥ 19

External signs appear when the nadis are pure. The body
will definitely be lean and bright.

यथेष्टं धारणं वायोरनलस्य प्रदीपनम् ।
नादाभिव्यक्तिरारोग्यं जायते नाडिशोधनात् ॥ 20

Retention of the breath as desired, stimulation of the digestion, manifestation of the nada, and good health come from purifying the nadis.

मेदश्लेष्माधिकः पूर्वं षट्कर्माणि समाचरेत् ।
अन्यस्तु नाचरेत्तानि दोषाणां समभावतः ॥ 21

One having too much fat and phlegm should first do the six karmans. But one who doesn't need not do them since his humors[4] are equable.

धौतिर्वस्तिस्तथा नेतिस्त्राटकं नौलिकं तथा ।
कपालभातिश्चैतानि षट्कर्माणि प्रचक्षते ॥ 22

These are the six karmans: Dhauti, Vasti, Neti, Trataka, Nauli, and Kapalabhati.

कर्मषट्कमिदं गोप्यं घटशोधनकारकम् ।
विचित्रगुणसंधायि पूज्यते योगिपुङ्गवैः ॥ 23

These six karmans—purifying the body, producing remarkable qualities—are to be given only to the worthy. They are honored by the best yogis.

चतुरङ्गुलविस्तारं हस्तपञ्चदशायतम् ।
गुरूपदिष्टमार्गेण सिक्तं वस्त्रं शनैर्ग्रसेत् ।

---

[4] Wind, bile, and phlegm.

पुनः प्रत्याहरेच्चैतदुदितं धौतिकर्म तत् ॥ 24

Slowly swallow a wet cloth which is four fingers wide and
fifteen hands long in the manner instructed by one's guru.
Draw it out again. This is called Dhautikarman.

कासश्वासप्लीहकुष्ठं कफरोगाश्च विंशतिः ।
धौतिकर्मप्रभावेण प्रयान्त्येव न संशयः ॥ 25

Coughing, asthma, enlargement of the spleen, leprosy,
and twenty other phlegm diseases vanish because of the
power of Dhautikarman. In this there is no doubt.

नाभिदघ्नजले पायौ न्यस्तनालोत्कटासनः ।
आधाराकुञ्चनं कुर्यात्क्षालनं वस्तिकर्म तत् ॥ 26

Assume Utkatasana in water as deep as the navel. Insert
a tube into the anus. Contract the anus. This cleansing
is Vastikarman.

गुल्मप्लीहोदरं चापि वातपित्तकफोद्भवाः ।
वस्तिकर्मप्रभावेण क्षीयन्ते सकलामयाः ॥ 27

Enlargements of the glands, spleen, and abdomen—and
all diseases arising from wind, bile, and phlegm—perish
due to the power of Vastikarman.

धात्विन्द्रियान्तःकरणप्रसादं दद्याच्च कान्तिं दहनप्रदीप्तिम् ।
अशेषदोषोपचयं निहन्यादभ्यस्यमानं जलवस्तिकर्म ॥ 28

Vastikarman in the water, when regularly practiced, gives clarity to the bodily constituents, the senses, and the mind. It gives luster to the body, stimulates the gastric fire, and eliminates all defects.

सूत्रं वितस्ति सुस्निग्धं नासानाले प्रवेशयेत् ।
मुखान्निर्गमयेच्चैषा नेतिः सिद्धैर्निगद्यते ॥ 29

Insert a very smooth thread nine inches long into a nasal passage and withdraw it from the mouth. This is called Neti by the masters.

कपालशोधिनी चैव दिव्यदृष्टिप्रदायिनी ।
जत्रूर्ध्वजातरोगौघं नेतिराशु निहन्ति च ॥ 30

Purifier of the skull and giver of divine sight, Neti quickly destroys the flood of diseases originating above the collarbone.

निरीक्षेन्निश्चलदृशा सूक्ष्मलक्ष्यं समाहितः ।
अश्रुसंपातपर्यन्तमाचार्यैस्त्राटकं स्मृतम् ॥ 31

Gaze with motionless eyes and concentration at a minute point until tears flow. This is called Trataka by gurus.

मोचनं नेत्ररोगाणां तन्द्रादीनां कपाटकम् ।
यत्नतस्त्राटकं गोप्यं यथा हाटकपेटकम् ॥ 32

Trataka removes eye diseases. It is a closed door to lethargy and so on. Strive to keep it secret—as if it were a gold box.

अमन्दावर्तवेगेन तुन्दं सव्यापसव्यतः ।
नतांसो भ्रामयेदेषा नौलिः सिद्धैः प्रचक्ष्यते ॥ 33

Lower the shoulders. Revolve the stomach left and right with the speed of a strong whirlpool. This is called Nauli by the masters.

मन्दाग्निसंदीपनपाचनादिसंधापिकानन्दकरी सदैव ।
अशेषदोषामयशोषणी च हठक्रियामौलिरियं च नौलिः ॥ 34

This Nauli is the crown of Hatha practices. It kindles a weak gastric fire, restores the digestion, etc., always brings happiness, and dries up all defects and diseases.

भस्त्रावलोहकारस्य रेचपूरौ ससंभ्रमौ ।
कपालभातिर्विख्याता कफदोषविशोषणी ॥ 35

Rapidly exhale and inhale like the bellows of a blacksmith. This is known as Kapalabhati. It dries up phlegm diseases.

षड्कर्मनिर्गतस्थौल्यकफदोषमलादिकः ।
प्राणायामं ततः कुर्यादनायासेन सिद्ध्यति ॥ 36

With fat, phlegm diseases, impurities, etc., removed by
the six karmans, one should then do pranayama. One will
succeed without strain.

प्राणायामैरेव सर्वे प्रशुष्यन्ति मला इति ।
आचार्याणां तु केषाञ्चिदन्यत्कर्म न संमतम् ॥ 37

"All impurities dry up by pranayama alone." Speaking thusly,
the other karmans are not approved of by some teachers.

उदरगतपदार्थमुद्धमन्ति पवनमपानमुदीर्य कण्ठनाले ।
क्रमपरिचयवश्यनाडिचक्रा गजकरणीति निगद्यते हठज्ञैः ॥ 38

Those who have the nadis under control from gradual
practice raise the apana wind in the esophagus and vomit
the stomach's contents. This is called Gajakarani by
knowers of Hatha.

ब्रह्मादयोऽपि त्रिदशाः पवनाभ्यासतत्पराः ।
अभूवन्नन्तकभयात्तस्मात्पवनमभ्यसेत् ॥ 39

Even Brahma and other gods engaged in pranayama
because they feared death. Therefore one should
practice pranayama.

यावद्बद्धो मरुद्देहे यावच्चित्तं निराकुलम् ।
यावद्दृष्टिर्भ्रुवोर्मध्ये तावत्कालभयं कुतः ॥ 40

As long as the breath is retained in the body, as long as the mind is calm, and as long as the sight is in the middle of the brows, where is the fear of death?

विधिवत्प्राणसंयामैनार्डीचक्रे विशोधिते ।
सुषुम्नावदनं भित्त्वा सुखाद्विशति मारुतः ॥ 41

The breath splits open the mouth of the Sushumna and enters easily once all the nadis are purified by restraining prana correctly.

मारुते मध्यसंचारे मनःस्थैर्यं प्रजायते ।
यो मनःसुस्थिरीभावः सैवावस्था मनोन्मनी ॥ 42

Steadiness of mind is born when the breath moves in the middle. This state of mental steadiness is manonmani.

तत्सिद्धये विधानज्ञाश्चित्रान्कुर्वन्ति कुम्भकान् ।
विचित्रकुम्भकाभ्यासाद्विचित्रां सिद्धिमाप्नुयात् ॥ 43

Those knowing the procedures do various kumbhakas to achieve it. From the practice of various kumbhakas, one obtains various powers.

सूर्यभेदनमुज्जायी सीत्कारी शीतली तथा ।
भस्त्रिका भ्रामरी मूर्च्छा प्लाविनीत्यष्टकुम्भकाः ॥ 44

These are the eight kumbhakas: Suryabhedana, Ujjayi, Sitkari, Shitali, Bhastrika, Bhramari, Murccha, and Plavini.

पूरकान्ते तु कर्तव्यो बन्धो जालन्धराभिधः ।
कुम्भकान्ते रेचकादौ कर्तव्यस्तूड्डियानकः ॥ 45

A bandha named Jalandhara is to be done at the end of inhalation. Uddiyana is to be done at the end of kumbhaka and the beginning of exhalation.

अधस्तात्कुञ्चनेनाशु कण्ठसंकोचने कृते ।
मध्ये पश्चिमतानेन स्यात्प्राणो ब्रह्मनाडिगः ॥ 46

The prana will enter the Brahma nadi when contraction of the throat,[5] contraction beneath,[6] and retraction in the middle[7] are done.

अपानमूर्ध्वमुत्थाप्य प्राणं कण्ठादधो नयेत् ।
योगी जराविमुक्तः सन्षोडशाब्दवयो भवेत् ॥ 47

Having raised the apana upwards, the yogi should guide the prana below the throat. Being liberated from old age, he will be a youth of sixteen.

आसने सुखदे योगी बद्ध्वा चैवासनं ततः ।
दक्षनाड्या समाकृष्य बहिःस्थं पवनं शनैः ॥ 48

Form an asana on a comfortable seat. Slowly draw in outside air through the right nadi.

---

[5] Jalandharabandha.
[6] Mulabandha.
[7] Uddiyanabandha.

आकेशादानखाग्राच्च निरोधावधि कुम्भयेत् ।
ततः शनैः सव्यनाड्या रेचयेत्पवनं शनैः ॥ 49

Form the kumbhaka to the limit—from the hair to the toenails. Exhale the breath very slowly through the left nadi.

कपालशोधनं वातदोषघ्नं कृमिदोषहृत् ।
पुनः पुनरिदं कार्यं सूर्यभेदनमुत्तमम् ॥ 50

This most excellent Suryabhedana is to be done again and again. It cleanses the skull, destroys wind diseases, and removes worm diseases.

मुखं संयम्य नाडीभ्यामाकृष्य पवनं शनैः ।
यथा लगति कण्ठात्तु हृदयावधि सस्वनम् ॥ 51
पूर्ववत्कुम्भयेत्प्राणं रेचयेदिडया ततः ।

Close the mouth. Slowly draw the breath through both nadis so it resonates from the throat to the heart. Form the kumbhaka as before. Exhale the prana through the Ida.

श्लेष्मदोषहरं कण्ठे देहानलविवर्धनम् ॥ 52
नाडीजलोदराधातुगतदोषविनाशनम् ।
गच्छता तिष्ठता कार्यमुज्जाय्याख्यं तु कुम्भकम् ॥ 53

This kumbhaka called Ujjayi can be done walking or standing. It removes phlegm diseases in the throat, increases digestive power in the body, and destroys dropsy and diseases of the nadis and of all bodily constituents.

सीत्कां कुर्यात्तथा वक्त्रे घ्राणेनैव विजृम्भिकाम् ।
एवमभ्यासयोगेन कामदेवो द्वितीयकः ॥ 54

Inhale making the sound "seet" in the mouth, then exhale only through the nose. By engaging in this practice one becomes a second God of Love.

योगिनीचक्रसामान्यः सृष्टिसंहारकारकः ।
न क्षुधा न तृषा निद्रा नैवालस्यं प्रजायते ॥ 55

Respected by all yoginis, maker of creation and destruction, neither hunger, nor thirst, nor sleep, nor even lethargy will appear.

भवेत्सत्त्वं च देहस्य सर्वोपद्रववर्जितः ।
अनेन विधिना सत्यं योगीन्द्रो भूमिमण्डले ॥ 56

This Sitkari will develop the body's vitality. The Lord of Yogis will be completely free of all disabilities on earth.

जिह्वया वायुमाकृष्य पूर्ववत्कुम्भसाधनम् ।
शनकैर्घ्राणरन्ध्राभ्यां रेचयेत्पवनं सुधीः ॥ 57

Draw in air with the tongue. Practice kumbhaka as before. Slowly exhale the air through the nostrils.

गुल्मप्लीहादिकान् रोगान् ज्वरं पित्तं क्षुधां तृषाम् ।
विषाणि शीतली नाम कुम्भिकेयं निहन्ति हि ॥ 58

This kumbhaka named Shitali destroys enlargement of
the glands or spleen, other diseases, fever, bile, hunger,
thirst, and poisons.

ऊर्वोरुपरि संस्थाप्य शुभे पादतले उभे ।
पद्मासनं भवेदेतत्सर्वपापप्रणाशनम् ॥ 59

Place both clean soles of the feet above the thighs. This is
Padmasana, destroyer of all evils.

सम्यक्पद्मासनं बद्ध्वा समग्रीवोदरं सुधीः ।
मुखं संयम्य यत्नेन प्राणं घ्राणेन रेचयेत् ॥ 60
यथा लगति हृत्कण्ठे कपालावधि सस्वनम् ।
वेगेन पूरयेच्चापि हृत्पद्मावधि मारुतम् ॥ 61

Form Padmasana correctly, neck and belly aligned.
Close the mouth. Expel the prana through the nose so it
resonates in the heart, throat, and up to the skull. Then
quickly inhale air up to the lotus of the heart.[8]

पुनर्विरेचयेत्तद्वत्पूरयेच्च पुनः पुनः ।
यथैव लोहकारेण भस्त्रा वेगेन चाल्यते ॥ 62
तथैव स्वशरीरस्थं चालयेत्पवनं धिया ।

---

[8] The Anahata chakra.

Exhale and inhale in the above manner again and again. Just as a blacksmith works the bellows with speed, move the breath in one's own body with the will.

यदा श्रमो भवेद्देहे तदा सूर्येण पूरयेत् ॥ 63
यथोदरं भवेत्पूर्णमनिलेन तथा लघु ।
धारयेन्नासिकां मध्यातर्जनीभ्यां विना दृढम् ॥ 64
विधिवत्कुम्भकं कृत्वा रेचयेदिडयानिलम् ।

When there is fatigue in the body, inhale through the sun and quickly fill the belly with air. Hold the nose firmly without the middle and index fingers. Do kumbhaka in the prescribed manner. Exhale the air through the Ida.

वातपित्तश्लेष्महरं शरीराग्निविवर्धनम् ॥ 65
कुण्डलीबोधकं क्षिप्रं पवनं सुखदं हितम् ।
ब्रह्मनाडीमुखे संस्थकफाद्यर्गलनाशनम् ॥ 66

This removes diseases of wind, bile, and phlegm. It increases the fire in the body and awakens the kundalini quickly. It purifies, gives pleasure, and is beneficial. It destroys the obstructions of phlegm, etc., that exist at the mouth of the Brahma nadi.

सम्यग्गात्रसमुद्भूतग्रन्थित्रयविभेदकम् ।
विशेषेणैव कर्तव्यं भस्त्राख्यं कुम्भकं त्विदम् ॥ 67

This kumbhaka called Bhastrika is to be done with great
regularity. It splits the three strong knots that form
in the body.

वेगाद्घोषं पूरकं भृङ्गनादं भृङ्गीनादं रेचकं मन्दमन्दम् ।
योगीन्द्राणामेवमभ्यासयोगाच्चित्ते जाता काचिदानन्दलीला ॥ 68

A quick and resonant inhalation sounding like a bee; a
very slow exhalation sounding like a female bee. Thus a
certain bliss and delight are born in the minds of good
yogis from doing Bhramari.

पूरकान्ते गाढतरं बद्ध्वा जालन्धरं शनैः ।
रेचयेन्मूर्च्छनाख्येयं मनोमूर्च्छा सुखप्रदा ॥ 69

At the end of inhalation, hold Jalandhara tightly and
slowly exhale. This one named Murccha clears the mind
and gives happiness.

अन्तःप्रवर्तितोदारमारुतापूरितोदरः ।
पयस्यगाधेऽपि सुखात्प्लवते पद्मपत्रवत् ॥ 70

Move a large amount of air inside, filling the belly. Float
happily like a lotus leaf, even in bottomless water.
This is Plavini.

प्राणायामस्त्रिधा प्रोक्तो रेचपूरककुम्भकैः ।
सहितः केवलश्चेति कुम्भको द्विविधो मतः ॥ 71

यावत्केवलसिद्धिः स्यात्सहितं तावदभ्यसेत् ।

Pranayama is said to be of three kinds: exhalation, inhalation, and kumbhaka. Kumbhaka is thought to be of two kinds—Sahita and Kevala. Until such time as Kevala is mastered, one should practice Sahita.

रेचकं पूरकं मुक्त्वा सुखं यद्वायुधारणम् ॥ 72
प्राणायामोऽयमित्युक्तः स वै केवलकुम्भकः ।

Abandon exhalation and inhalation. Hold the breath comfortably. This pranayama is the one called Kevalakumbhaka.

कुम्भके केवले सिद्धे रेचपूरकवर्जिते ॥ 73
न तस्य दुर्लभं किंचित्त्रिषु लोकेषु विद्यते ।

Nothing in the three worlds is hard to win by one who masters Kevalakumbhaka without exhalation or inhalation.

शक्तः केवलकुम्भेन यथेष्टं वायुधारणात् ॥ 74
राजयोगपदं चापि लभते नात्र संशयः ।

One made powerful by Kevalakumbhaka, from holding the breath as desired, obtains even the state of Raja Yoga. In this there is no doubt.

कुम्भकात्कुण्डलीबोधः कुण्डलीबोधतो भवेत् ॥ 75
अनर्गला सुषुम्ना च हठसिद्धिश्च जायते ।

Through kumbhaka, the kundalini is awakened. Through awakening the kundalini, the Sushumna is unblocked— and success in Hatha is born.

हठं विना राजयोगो राजयोगं विना हठः ।
न सिध्यति ततो युग्ममानिष्पत्तेः समभ्यसेत् ॥ 76

Raja Yoga will not be complete without Hatha, nor Hatha without Raja Yoga. Therefore practice the pair to perfection.

कुम्भकप्राणरोधान्ते कुर्याच्चित्तं निराश्रयम् ।
एवमभ्यासयोगेन राजयोगपदं व्रजेत् ॥ 77

Make the mind without objects at the end of the retention of the prana in kumbhaka. One should reach the state of Raja Yoga by engaging in this practice.

वपुःकृशत्वं वदने प्रसन्नता नादस्फुटत्वं नयने सुनिर्मले ।
अरोगता बिन्दुजयोऽग्निदीपनं नाडीविशुद्धिर्हठसिद्धिलक्षणम् ॥ 78

These are indicators of success in Hatha: leanness of body, clearness of face, distinctness of nada, very clear eyes, health, victory over bindu, lighting of the digestive fire, and purity of the nadis.

इति हठयोगप्रदीपिकायां द्वितीयोपदेशः ॥

Thus ends the second chapter in the Hatha Yoga Pradipika.

Chapter Three

Mudras

सशैलवनधात्रीणां यथाधारोऽहिनायकः ।
सर्वेषां योगतन्त्राणां तथाधारो हि कुण्डली ॥ 1

As the Lord of Serpents supports the earth with its mountains and forests, so kundalini supports all Yoga practices.

सुप्ता गुरुप्रसादेन यदा जागर्ति कुण्डली ।
तदा सर्वाणि पद्मानि भिद्यन्ते ग्रन्थयोऽपि च ॥ 2

All lotuses[1] and knots are split open when the sleeping kundalini is awakened by the grace of a guru.

प्राणस्य शून्यपदवी तदा राजपथायते ।
तदा चित्तं निरालम्बं तदा कालस्य वञ्चनम् ॥ 3

Then the cleared path[2] becomes the royal road for prana. Then the mind is without objects. Then death is tricked.

---

[1] Chakras.
[2] Sushumna.

सुषुम्ना शून्यपदवी ब्रह्मरन्ध्रं महापथः ।
श्मशानं शाम्भवी मध्यमार्गश्चेत्येकवाचकाः ॥ 4

Sushumna, Shunyapadavi, Brahmarandhra, Mahapatha,
Shmashana, Shambhavi, and Madhyamarga are synonyms.

तस्मात्सर्वप्रयत्नेन प्रबोधयितुमीश्वरीम् ।
ब्रह्मद्वारमुखे सुप्तां मुद्राभ्यासं समाचरेत् ॥ 5

Therefore practice mudras energetically to awaken the
goddess sleeping outside the door to Brahman.

महामुद्रा महाबन्धो महावेधश्च खेचरी ।
उड्डयानं मूलबन्धश्च बन्धो जालन्धराभिधः ॥ 6
करणी विपरीताख्या वज्रोली शक्तिचालनम् ।
इदं हि मुद्रादशकं जरामरणनाशनम् ॥ 7

These are the ten mudras which together destroy old
age and death: Mahamudra, Mahabandha, Mahavedha,
Khechari, Uddiyana, Mulabandha, Jalandharabandha,
Viparitakarani, Vajroli, and Shaktichalana.

आदिनाथोदितं दिव्यमष्टैश्वर्यप्रदायकम् ।
वल्लभं सर्वसिद्धानां दुर्लभं मरुतामपि ॥ 8

These were taught by Shiva. They are divine, cherished
by all masters, hard to attain even by the gods, and give
the eight powers.

गोपनीयं प्रयत्नेन यथा रत्नकरण्डकम् ।
कस्यचिन्नैव वक्तव्यं कुलस्त्रीसुरतं यथा ॥ ९

Strive to keep them secret, as if they were a box of jewels.
Like sex with a respectable woman, don't talk about
them to anyone.

पादमूलेन वामेन योनिं संपीड्य दक्षिणम् ।
प्रसारितं पदं कृत्वा कराभ्यां धारयेद्दृढम् ॥ १०
कण्ठे बन्धं समारोप्य धारयेद्वायुमूर्ध्वतः ।

Press the perineum with the root of the left foot. Stretch
out the right foot and hold it firmly with both hands.
Form a bandha in the throat. Hold the breath high.

यथा दण्डहतः सर्पो दण्डाकारः प्रजायते ॥ ११
ऋज्वीभूता तथा शक्तिः कुण्डली सहसा भवेत् ।
तदा सा मरणावस्था जायते द्विपुटाश्रया ॥ १२

As a snake hit with a stick assumes the shape of a stick, so
the kundalini power will immediately straighten. Then a
state of death occurs in the two sides.[3]

ततः शनैः शनैरेव रेचयेन्नैव वेगतः ।
इयं खलु महामुद्रा महासिद्धैः प्रदर्शिता ॥ १३

Then exhale very slowly—never quickly. This is certainly
the Mahamudra shown by the great masters.

---

[3] In Ida and Pingala.

महाक्लेशादयो दोषाः क्षीयन्ते मरणादयः ।
महामुद्रां च तेनैव वदन्ति विबुधोत्तमाः ॥ 14

Great troubles, defects, death, and so on are eliminated.
The wisest of men call it Mahamudra for this very reason.

चन्द्राङ्घ्रे तु समभ्यस्य सूर्याङ्घ्रे पुनरभ्यसेत् ।
यावत्तुल्या भवेत्संख्या ततो मुद्रां विसर्जयेत् ॥ 15

After practicing on the moon side, practice again on the
sun side. Release the mudra when the number is equal.

न हि पथ्यमपथ्यं वा रसाः सर्वेऽपि नीरसाः ।
अपि भुक्तं विषं घोरं पीयूषमिव जीर्यति ॥ 16

There is neither prescribed nor prohibited food. All drinks
are digested like nectar, even if foul or a horrible poison.

क्षयकुष्ठगुदावर्तगुल्माजीर्णपुरोगमाः ।
तस्य दोषाः क्षयं यान्ति महामुद्रां तु योऽभ्यसेत् ॥ 17

The diseases of consumption, leprosy, constipation,
enlargement of the glands, indigestion, etc., disappear
when one practices Mahamudra.

कथितेयं महामुद्रा महासिद्धिकरी नृणाम् ।
गोपनीया प्रयत्नेन न देया यस्य कस्यचित् ॥ 18

This Mahamudra just described gives people great powers. It should be carefully kept secret and not given to just anyone.

पार्ष्णिं वामस्य पादस्य योनिस्थाने नियोजयेत् ।
वामोरूपरि संस्थाप्य दक्षिणं चरणं तथा ॥ 19

Place the right foot above the left thigh. Join the heel of the left foot to the perineum.

पूरयित्वा ततो वायुं हृदये चिबुकं दृढम् ।
निष्पीड्य योनिमाकुञ्ज्य मनो मध्ये नियोजयेत् ॥ 20

Then inhale air. Press the chin firmly on the heart. Contract the anus. Join the mind in the middle.

धारयित्वा यथाशक्ति रेचयेदनिलं शनैः ।
सव्याङ्गे तु समभ्यस्य दक्षाङ्गे पुनरभ्यसेत् ॥ 21

Hold as long as possible. Exhale the breath slowly. Having practiced on the left side, practice again on the right side.

मतमत्र तु केषाञ्चित्कण्ठबन्धं विवर्जयेत् ।
राजदन्तस्थजिह्वायां बन्धः शस्तो भवेदिति ॥ 22
अयं तु सर्वनाडीनामूर्ध्वगतिनिरोधकः ।

The opinion of some in this matter: "Avoid the throat contraction. Contact of the tongue on the front teeth is proper." This obstructs the upward motion of all the nadis.

अयं खलु महाबन्धो महासिद्धिप्रदायकः ॥ 23
कालपाशमहाबन्धविमोचनविचक्षणः ।
त्रिवेणीसङ्गमं धत्ते केदारं प्रापयेन्मनः ॥ 24

This Mahabandha is indeed the giver of great powers, clever in loosening the great noose of the rope of time. It creates the confluence of the three streams. It causes the mind to reach Kedara.[4]

रूपलावण्यसंपन्ना यथा स्त्री पुरुषं विना ।
महामुद्रामहाबन्धौ निष्फलौ वेधवर्जितौ ॥ 25

As a beautiful and charming woman without a man, so Mahamudra and Mahabandha are pointless without Mahavedha.

महाबन्धस्थितो योगी कृत्वा पूरकमेकधीः ।
वायूनां गतिमावृत्य निभृतं कण्ठमुद्रया ॥ 26

Assume Mahabandha, inhale, and maintain a one-pointed mind. Turn the motion of the breath into stillness with the throat mudra.

---

[4] A mountain in the Himalayas where Shiva resides. Also the place between the brows.

समहस्तयुगो भूमौ स्फिचौ संताडयेच्छनैः ।
पुटद्वयमतिक्रम्य वायुः स्फुरति मध्यगः ॥ 27

Place both hands flat on the ground. Slowly strike the
buttocks on the ground. The breath quivers after leaving
the two sides and entering the middle.

सोमसूर्याग्निसंबन्धो जायते चामृताय वै ।
मृतावस्था समुत्पन्ना ततो वायुं विरेचयेत् ॥ 28

This fusion of moon, sun, and fire[5] surely results in immortality. A state like death arises. Then exhale the breath.

महावेधोऽयमभ्यासान्महासिद्धिप्रदायकः ।
वलीपलितवेपघ्नः सेव्यते साधकोत्तमैः ॥ 29

This Mahavedha gives great powers with regular practice.
It kills wrinkles, gray hair, and trembling. It is practiced
by the best aspirants.

एतत्त्रयं महागुह्यं जरामृत्युविनाशनम् ।
वह्निवृद्धिकरं चैव ह्याणिमादिगुणप्रदम् ॥ 30

These three should be kept a great secret. They destroy
old age and death, increase the digestive fire, and give
qualities like animan.[6]

---

[5] The three streams—Ida, Pingala, and Sushumna.
[6] The ability to make oneself very small.

अष्टधा क्रियते चैव यामे यामे दिने दिने ।
पुण्यसंभारसंधायि पापौघविभिदुरं सदा ।
सम्यक्शिक्षावतामेवं स्वल्पं प्रथमसाधनम् ॥ 31

They are to be done eight times every day, every three
hours, with few repetitions in the beginning. They give a
wealth of merit and always destroy a heap of sins for those
who receive proper instruction.

कपालकुहरे जिह्वा प्रविष्टा विपरीतगा ।
भ्रुवोरन्तर्गता दृष्टिर्मुद्रा भवति खेचरी ॥ 32

Turn the tongue backward and insert it into the skull
cavity. Direct the gaze to the middle of the brows. This
is Khecharimudra.

छेदनचालनदोहैः कलां क्रमेण वर्धयेत्तावत् ।
सा यावद्भ्रूमध्यं स्पृशति तदा खेचरीसिद्धिः ॥ 33

Gradually elongate the tongue by cutting, shaking, and
stretching it until it touches the middle of the brows.
Then Khechari is accomplished.

स्नुहीपत्रनिभं शस्त्रं सुतीक्ष्णं स्निग्धनिर्मलम् ।
समादाय ततस्तेन रोममात्रं समुच्छिनेत् ॥ 34

Take a smooth, stainless knife—very sharp, like a snuhi
leaf—and cut a hair's breadth with it.

ततः सैन्धवपथ्याभ्यां चूर्णिताभ्यां प्रधर्षयेत् ।
पुनः सप्तदिने प्राप्ते रोममात्रं समुच्छिनेत् ॥ 35

Then rub it with a powder of rock salt and yellow
myrobalan. When the seventh day arrives, cut a hair's
breadth again.

एवं क्रमेण षण्मासं नित्यं युक्तः समाचरेत् ।
षण्मासाद्रसनामूलशिराबन्धः प्रणश्यति ॥ 36

Practice regularly in this manner for six months. The tie
of blood vessel at the root of the tongue disappears after
six months.

कलां पराङ्मुखीं कृत्वा त्रिपथे परियोजयेत् ।
सा भवेत्खेचरी मुद्रा व्योमचक्रं तदुच्यते ॥ 37

Turn the tongue backward and insert it into the path of
the three. This is Khecharimudra. It is also called
Vyomachakra.

रसनामूर्ध्वगां कृत्वा क्षणार्धमपि तिष्ठति ।
विषैर्विमुच्यते योगी व्याधिमृत्युजरादिभिः ॥ 38

The yogi who holds the tongue upward for even half a
second is saved from poison, disease, death, old age,
and so on.

न रोगो मरणं तन्द्रा न निद्रा न क्षुधा तृषा ।
न च मूर्च्छा भवेत्तस्य यो मुद्रां वेत्ति खेचरीम् ॥ ३९

He who knows Khecharimudra is without disease, death, lethargy, sleep, hunger, thirst, and fainting.

पीड्यते न स रोगेण लिप्यते न च कर्मणा ।
बाध्यते न स कालेन यो मुद्रां वेत्ति खेचरीम् ॥ ४०

He who knows Khecharimudra is not tormented by disease, not smeared with Karma, not troubled by time.

चित्तं चरति खे यस्माज्जिह्वा चरति खे गता ।
तेनैषा खेचरी नाम मुद्रा सिद्धैर्निरूपिता ॥ ४१

The mind moves in space; the tongue enters space. Therefore the name Khechari[7] was chosen by the masters for this mudra.

खेचर्या मुद्रितं येन विवरं लम्बिकोर्ध्वतः ।
न तस्य क्षरते बिन्दुः कामिन्याः श्लेषितस्य च ॥ ४२

The semen does not flow (even when embraced by a passionate woman) if the cavity above the soft palate is sealed with the Khechari.

चलितोऽपि यदा बिन्दुः संप्राप्तो योनिमण्डलम् ।

---

[7] Kha means space and chari means to move.

व्रजत्यूर्ध्वं हतः शक्त्या निबद्धो योनिमुद्रया ॥ 43

Even when the semen flows and reaches the region of the penis, it is arrested by the Yonimudra[8] and carried forcibly upward.

ऊर्ध्वजिह्वः स्थिरो भूत्वा सोमपानं करोति यः ।
मासार्धेन न संदेहो मृत्युं जयति योगवित् ॥ 44

The knower of Yoga—tongue above, steady, drinking soma[9]—undoubtedly conquers death in half a month.

नित्यं सोमकलापूर्णं शरीरं यस्य योगिनः ।
तक्षकेणापि दष्टस्य विषं तस्य न सर्पति ॥ 45

Poison does not spread in the yogi whose body is filled every day with drops of soma—even when bitten by the Takshaka serpent.

इन्धनानि यथा वह्निस्तैलवर्तिं च दीपकः ।
तथा सोमकलापूर्णं देही देहं न मुञ्चति ॥ 46

As the fire, the fuel, and the flame, the oily wick, so the soul does not abandon a body filled with drops of soma.

गोमांसं भक्षयेन्नित्यं पिबेदमरवारुणीम् ।

---

[8] Vajrolimudra.
[9] Drops that fall from the cavity above the palate.

कुलीनं तमहं मन्ये चेतरे कुलघातकाः ॥ 47

I regard one who would eat cow meat and drink divine liquor every day to be well born. Others destroy the family.

गोशब्देनोदिता जिह्वा तत्प्रवेशो हि तालुनि ।
गोमांसभक्षणं तत्तु महापातकनाशनम् ॥ 48

The word "cow" means tongue. Its insertion into the palate is "eating cow meat." This destroys the five great sins.

जिह्वाप्रवेशसंभूतवह्निनोत्पादितः खलु ।
चन्द्रात्स्रवति यः सारः सा स्यादमरवारुणी ॥ 49

"Divine liquor" is the essence that flows from the moon. It is produced by the fire born of the insertion of the tongue.

चुम्बन्ती यदि लम्बिकाग्रमनिशं जिह्वा रसस्यन्दिनी
सक्षारा कटुकाम्लदुग्धसदृशी मध्वाज्यतुल्या तथा ।
व्याधीनां हरणं जरान्तकरणं शस्त्रागमोदीरणं
तस्य स्यादमरत्वमष्टगुणितं सिद्धाङ्गनाकर्षणम् ॥ 50

If the tongue continuously touches the tip of the soft palate, making the juice flow—salty, pungent, sour, similar to milk, the same as honey and ghee—then these will be his: destruction of diseases, the end of old age, deflection of the onslaught of weapons, immortality, the eight siddhis, and attraction of the siddhas' women.

मूर्ध्नः षोडशपत्रपद्मगलितं प्राणाद्वाप्तं हठा-
दूर्ध्वास्यो रसनां नियम्य विवरे शक्तिं परां चिन्तयन् ।
उत्कल्लोलकलाजलं च विमलं धारामयं यः पिबे-
न्निर्व्याधिः स मृणालकोमलवपुर्योगी चिरं जीवति ॥ 51

The yogi who turns the face upward,[10] holds the tongue in the cavity, meditates upon the highest shakti, and drinks the clear stream of flooding crescent water—flowing from the head to the sixteen-petaled lotus,[11] obtained from prana and Hatha—that yogi lives long and without disease, body soft as the root of a lotus.

यत्प्रालेयं प्रहितसुषिरं मेरुमूर्धान्तरस्थं
तस्मिंस्तत्त्वं प्रवदति सुधीस्तन्मुखं निम्नगानाम् ।
चन्द्रात्सारः स्रवति वपुषस्तेन मृत्युर्नराणां
तद्बध्नीयात्सुकरणमथो नान्यथा कायसिद्धिः ॥ 52

The wise man considers the dew flowing from the cavity within Meru's summit to be Reality. It is the mouth of all rivers. Men die when the body's essence flows from the moon. Therefore form the good device.[12] Otherwise there is no perfection of the body.

---

[10] Who assumes Viparitakarani.
[11] Vishuddhi chakra.
[12] Khecharimudra.

सुषिरं ज्ञानजनकं पञ्चस्रोतःसमन्वितम् ।
तिष्ठते खेचरी मुद्रा तस्मिञ्छून्ये निरञ्जने ॥ 53

The cavity, a generator of wisdom, is united with the
five streams. In that unstained emptiness stands
Khecharimudra.

एकं सृष्टिमयं बीजमेका मुद्रा च खेचरी ।
एको देवो निरालम्ब एकावस्था मनोन्मनी ॥ 54

There is only one seed,[13] pervading creation; one mudra,
Khechari; one God, independent; one state, manonmani.

बद्धो येन सुषुम्नायां प्राणस्तूड्डीयते यतः ।
तस्मादुड्डीयनाख्योऽयं योगिभिः समुदाहृतः ॥ 55

This is called Uddiyana[14] by the yogis because the prana
is bound and flies up the Sushumna.

उड्डीनं कुरुते यस्मादविश्रान्तं महाखगः ।
उड्डीयानं तदेव स्यात्तत्र बन्धोऽभिधीयते ॥ 56

Only the one inducing the great bird[15] to fly up without a
break is Uddiyana. Now the bandha is explained.

उदरे पश्चिमं तानं नाभेरूर्ध्वं च कारयेत् ।

---

[13] Bijakshara, or ॐ.
[14] Ud means upward and di means to fly.
[15] Prana.

उड्डीयानो ह्यसौ बन्धो मृत्युमातङ्गकेसरी ॥ 57

Draw the belly backward and the navel upward. This Uddiyanabandha is surely the lion that kills the elephant of death.

उड्डीयानं तु सहजं गुरुणा कथितं यदा ।
अभ्यसेत्सततं यस्तु वृद्धोऽपि तरुणायते ॥ 58

One who constantly practices Uddiyana as described by a guru until it is natural becomes young, even if old.

नाभेरूर्ध्वमधश्चापि तानं कुर्यात्प्रयत्नतः ।
षण्मासमभ्यसेन्मृत्युं जयत्येव न संशयः ॥ 59

Draw in above and below the navel. Practice diligently for six months. Then one conquers death without a doubt.

सर्वेषामेव बन्धानामुत्तमो ह्युड्डियानकः ।
उड्डियाने दृढे बन्धे मुक्तिः स्वाभाविकी भवेत् ॥ 60

Uddiyana is definitely the best of all the bandhas. Liberation will be natural once Uddiyanabandha is mastered.

पार्ष्णिभागेन संपीड्य योनिमाकुञ्चयेद्गुदम् ।
अपानमूर्ध्वमाकृष्य मूलबन्धोऽभिधीयते ॥ 61

Press the perineum with the heel. Contract the anus. Draw the apana upwards. This is called Mulabandha.

अधोगतिमपानं वा ऊर्ध्वगं कुरुते बलात् ।
आकुञ्चनेन तं प्राहुर्मूलबन्धं हि योगिनः ॥ 62

One makes the apana, which goes downward, go upward by contracting forcefully. Yogis call that Mulabandha.[16]

गुदं पाष्ण्र्या तु संपीड्य वायुमाकुञ्चयेद्बलात् ।
वारं वारं यथा चोर्ध्वं समायाति समीरणः ॥ 63

Press the anus with the heel. Compress the breath forcefully again and again so it goes upwards.

प्राणापानौ नादबिन्दू मूलबन्धेन चैकताम् ।
गत्वा योगस्य संसिद्धिं यच्छतो नात्र संशयः ॥ 64

Prana and apana, and nada and bindu, give success in Yoga after they are united by Mulabandha. Here there is no doubt.

अपानप्राणयोरैक्यं क्षयो मूत्रपुरीषयोः ।
युवा भवति वृद्धोऽपि सततं मूलबन्धनात् ॥ 65

---

[16] It is called Mulabandha because the Muladhara chakra is contracted.

Prana and apana unite, urine and excrement decline, even
the old become young—all from the regular practice
of Mulabandha.

अपाने ऊर्ध्वगे जाते प्रयाते वह्निमण्डलम् ।
तदानलशिखा दीर्घा जायते वायुनाहता ॥ 66

The gastric flames shoot higher when the apana ascends
and strikes the sphere of fire.[17]

ततो यातो वह्न्यपानौ प्राणमुष्णस्वरूपकम् ।
तेनात्यन्तप्रदीप्तस्तु ज्वलनो देहजस्तथा ॥ 67

Then the gastric fire and the apana join the prana, which
is naturally hot, and the body's fire is stoked.

तेन कुण्डलिनी सुप्ता संतप्ता संप्रबुध्यते ।
दण्डाहता भुजङ्गीव निश्वस्य ऋजुतां व्रजेत् ॥ 68

Due to this heat the sleeping kundalini is awakened,
hissing and straightening like a snake struck by a stick.

बिलं प्रविष्टेव ततो ब्रह्मनाड्यन्तरं व्रजेत् ।
तस्मान्नित्यं मूलबन्धः कर्तव्यो योगिभिः सदा ॥ 69

---

[17] Located below the navel.

Then it goes into the Brahma nadi like a snake entering its hole. Therefore yogis should always do Mulabandha every day.

कण्ठमाकुञ्ज्य हृदये स्थापयेच्चिबुकं दृढम् ।
बन्धो जालन्धराख्योऽयं जरामृत्युविनाशकः ॥ 70

After contracting the throat, place the chin firmly on the heart. This is called Jalandharabandha. It destroys old age and death.

बध्नाति हि सिराजालमधोगामि नभोजलम् ।
ततो जालन्धरो बन्धः कण्ठदुःखौघनाशनः ॥ 71

It binds the web of nadis and halts the downward course of the water of the sky. Thus Jalandharabandha.[18] It destroys the flood of maladies of the throat.

जालन्धरे कृते बन्धे कण्ठसंकोचलक्षणे ।
न पीयूषं पतत्यग्नौ न च वायुः प्रकुप्यति ॥ 72

The nectar does not fall into the digestive fire and the breath is not malevolent when Jalandharabandha, whose mark is contraction of the throat, is done.

कण्ठसंकोचनेनैव द्वे नाड्यौ स्तम्भयेद्दृढम् ।

---

[18] Jalandhara means both "one that holds the web of nadis" and "one that holds the water of the cavity."

मध्यचक्रमिदं ज्ञेयं षोडशाधारबन्धनम् ॥ 73

The two nadis are firmly bound just by contracting the throat. This should be known as the middle chakra,[19] which binds the sixteen adharas.[20]

मूलस्थानं समाकुञ्च्य उड्डियानं तु कारयेत् ।
इडां च पिङ्गलां बद्ध्वा वाहयेत्पश्चिमे पथि ॥ 74

Contract the anus. Do Uddiyana. Bind Ida and Pingala. Make the breath flow into the hind path.[21]

अनेनैव विधानेन प्रयाति पवनो लयम् ।
ततो न जायते मृत्युर्जरारोगादिकं तथा ॥ 75

This is the way the breath becomes absorbed. Then there is no death, old age, disease, and so on.

बन्धत्रयमिदं श्रेष्ठं महासिद्धैश्च सेवितम् ।
सर्वेषां हठतन्त्राणां साधनं योगिनो विदुः ॥ 76

This triad of bandhas is the best. It is practiced by the great masters. Yogis know it accomplishes all Hatha practices.

यत्किंचित्स्रवते चन्द्रादमृतं दिव्यरूपिणः ।
तत्सर्वं ग्रसते सूर्यस्तेन पिण्डो जरायुतः ॥ 77

---

[19] Vishuddhi.
[20] Regions in the body.
[21] Sushumna.

Whatever nectar flows from the moon (whose form is divine) is swallowed by the sun. Consequently the body ages.

तत्रास्ति करणं दिव्यं सूर्यस्य मुखवञ्चनम् ।
गुरूपदेशतो ज्ञेयं न तु शास्त्रार्थकोटिभिः ॥ 78

There is a divine act that tricks the mouth of the sun. It is learned from a guru's instruction, not from crores[22] of explications of the Shastras.

ऊर्ध्वनाभेरधस्तालोरूर्ध्वं भानुरधः शशी ।
करणी विपरीताख्या गुरुवाक्येन लभ्यते ॥ 79

Navel above, palate below, sun above, moon below— this is called Viparitakarani.[23] It is obtained from a guru's instruction.

नित्यमभ्यासयुक्तस्य जठराग्निविवर्धिनी ।
आहारो बहुलस्तस्य संपाद्यः साधकस्य च ॥ 80
अल्पाहारो यदि भवेदग्निर्दहति तत्क्षणात् ।

Daily practice increases the stomach's fire, so the practitioner should have plenty of food. If he eats too little food, the fire burns him instantly.

---

[22] One crore equals ten million.
[23] Probably the same as Sarvangasana.

अधःशिराश्रोर्ध्वपादः क्षणं स्यात्प्रथमे दिने ॥ 81
क्षणाञ्च किंचिदधिकमभ्यसेञ्च दिने दिने ।

Hold the head down and the feet up for just a moment on
the first day. Practice it longer and longer every day.

वलितं पलितं चैव षण्मासोर्ध्वं न दृश्यते ।
याममात्रं तु यो नित्यमभ्यसेत्स तु कालजित् ॥ 82

Wrinkles and gray hair are invisible after just six months.
He who practices it for three hours every day surely
conquers death.

स्वेच्छया वर्तमानोऽपि योगोक्तैर्नियमैर्विना ।
वज्रोलीं यो विजानाति स योगी सिद्धिभाजनम् ॥ 83

The yogi who knows Vajroli receives powers even when
living without inhibitions or the observances spoken
of by Yoga.

तत्र वस्तुद्वयं वक्ष्ये दुर्लभं यस्य कस्यचित् ।
क्षीरं चैकं द्वितीयं तु नारी च वशवर्तिनी ॥ 84

For this I will list two items not everyone can obtain: one
is milk,[24] the second is a female partner.

मेहनेन शनैः सम्यगूर्ध्वाकुञ्चनमभ्यसेत् ।

---

[24] For drinking after intercourse.

पुरुषोऽप्यथवा नारी वज्रोलीसिद्धिमाप्नुयात् ॥ 85

Slowly and carefully practice drawing upward when the semen flows. A man, or even a woman, will obtain success in Vajroli.

यत्नतः शस्तनालेन फूत्कारं वज्रकन्दरे ।
शनैः शनैः प्रकुर्वीत वायुसंचारकारणात् ॥ 86

Blow firmly and very slowly into the hole of the thunderbolt with a suitable hollow stalk to allow air movement.

नारीभगे पतद्विन्दुमभ्यासेनोर्ध्वमाहरेत् ।
चलितं च निजं बिन्दुमूर्ध्वमाकृष्य रक्षयेत् ॥ 87

Practice bringing upward the semen that is falling into the woman's genital organ. Draw up and preserve one's own flowing semen.

एवं संरक्षयेद्विन्दुं मृत्युं जयति योगवित् ।
मरणं बिन्दुपातेन जीवनं बिन्दुधारणात् ॥ 88

The knower of Yoga should preserve his semen and thereby conquer death. Emission of semen is death; preservation of semen is life.

सुगन्धो योगिनो देहे जायते बिन्दुधारणात् ।
यावद्विन्दुः स्थिरो देहे तावत्कालभयं कुतः ॥ 89

Preservation of semen produces a good fragrance in the body of the yogi. As long as the semen is firmly in the body, where is the fear of death?

चित्तायत्तं नृणां शुक्रं शुक्रायत्तं च जीवितम् ।
तस्माच्छुक्रं मनश्चैव रक्षणीयं प्रयत्नतः ॥ 90

Life depends on semen, and men's semen depends on the mind. Therefore vigorously protect both semen and mind.

ऋतुमत्या रजोऽप्येवं निजं बिन्दुं च रक्षयेत् ।
मेण्ढ्रेणाकर्षयेदूर्ध्वं सम्यगभ्यासयोगवित् ॥ 91

Thus the knower of this Yoga practice should draw upwards with the penis to preserve his own semen and even the seminal fluid of a woman who has just completed menstruation.

सहजोलिश्चामरोलिर्वज्रोल्या भेद एकतः ।
जले सुभस्म निक्षिप्य दग्धगोमयसंभवम् ॥ 92
वज्रोलीमैथुनादूर्ध्वं स्त्रीपुंसोः स्वाङ्गलेपनम् ।
आसीनयोः सुखेनैव मुक्तव्यापारयोः क्षणात् ॥ 93

Sahajoli and Amaroli are equivalent types of Vajroli. Put good ashes made of burnt cow dung in water. After copulating in Vajroli—just sitting happily, their embrace released pleasurably—a man and woman should smear their important parts.

सहजोलिरियं प्रोक्ता श्रद्धेया योगिभिः सदा ।
अयं शुभकरो योगो भोगयुक्तोऽपि मुक्तिदः ॥ 94

This is called Sahajoli. Yogis can always count on it. This
auspicious yoga, even though mixed with pleasure,
gives liberation.

अयं योगः पुण्यवतां धीराणां तत्त्वदर्शिनाम् ।
निर्मत्सराणां वै सिध्येन्न तु मत्सरशालिनाम् ॥ 95

The meritorious, the brave, realists, and those free from
envy will succeed at this yoga—but not the envious.

पित्तोल्बणत्वात्प्रथमाम्बुधारां विहाय निःसारतयान्त्यधाराम् ।
निषेव्यते शीतलमध्यधारा कापालिके खण्डमतेऽमरोली ॥ 96

Discard the beginning of the stream of water because it
has too much bile. Discard the end of the stream because
it is worthless. Wholly enjoy the cool, middle stream.
This is Amaroli in the opinion of the Khandakapalikas.[25]

अमरीं यः पिबेन्नित्यं नस्यं कुर्वन्दिने दिने ।
वज्रोलीमभ्यसेत्सम्यक्सामरोलीति कथ्यते ॥ 97

One who drinks amari every day by drawing it through
the nose practices Vajroli correctly. This is called Amaroli.

---

[25] A Shaiva sect.

अभ्यासान्निःसृतां चान्द्रीं विभूत्या सह मिश्रयेत् ।
धारयेदुत्तमाङ्गेषु दिव्यदृष्टिः प्रजायते ॥ 98

Mix the lunar nectar released by this practice with
cow-dung ashes and smear one's important parts. Divine
sight is born.

पुंसो बिन्दुं समाकुञ्च्य सम्यगभ्यासपाटवात् ।
यदि नारी रजो रक्षेद्वज्रोल्या सापि योगिनी ॥ 99

If a woman, with expertise from proper practice, draws
up the semen of a man and preserves her seminal fluid
with Vajroli, then she, too, is a yogini.

तस्याः किंचिद्रजो नाशं न गच्छति न संशयः ।
तस्याः शरीरे नादश्च बिन्दुतामेव गच्छति ॥ 100

Without a doubt, not a bit of her seminal fluid is lost.
Nada definitely reaches bindu in her body.

स बिन्दुस्तद्रजश्चैव एकीभूय स्वदेहगौ ।
वज्रोल्यभ्यासयोगेन सर्वसिद्धिं प्रयच्छतः ॥ 101

The semen and the seminal fluid, combined in one's own
body by the practice of Vajroli, give all powers.

रक्षेदाकुञ्चनादूर्ध्वं या रजः सा हि योगिनी ।
अतीतानागतं वेत्ति खेचरी च भवेद्ध्रुवम् ॥ 102

She who preserves her seminal fluid by drawing upwards is indeed a yogini. She knows the past and the future, and surely moves in the sky.

देहसिद्धिं च लभते वज्रोल्यभ्यासयोगतः ।
अयं पुण्यकरो योगो भोगे भुक्तेऽपि मुक्तिदः ॥ 103

One obtains bodily perfection by practicing Vajroli. This yoga produces merit and gives liberation even though pleasure is enjoyed.

कुटिलाङ्गी कुण्डलिनी भुजङ्गी शक्तिरीश्वरी ।
कुण्डल्यरुन्धती चैते शब्दाः पर्यायवाचकाः ॥ 104

Kutilangi, kundalini, bhujangi, shakti, ishvari, kundali, and arundhati—these words are synonyms.

उद्घाटयेत्कपाटं तु यथा कुञ्चिकया हठात् ।
कुण्डलिन्या तथा योगी मोक्षद्वारं विभेदयेत् ॥ 105

As one opens a door with a key, so the yogi opens the door of liberation with Hatha's kundalini.

येन मार्गेण गन्तव्यं ब्रह्मस्थानं निरामयम् ।
मुखेनाच्छाद्य तद्द्वारं प्रसुप्ता परमेश्वरी ॥ 106

Kundalini sleeps with her mouth covering the entrance to the path that leads to the region of Brahman, which is free of disease.

कन्दोर्ध्व कुण्डली शक्तिः सुप्ता मोक्षाय योगिनाम् ।
बन्धनाय च मूढानां यस्तां वेत्ति स योगवित् ॥ 107

Kundalini, sleeping above the kanda, liberates yogis and binds the ignorant. He who knows her, knows Yoga.

कुण्डली कुटिलाकारा सर्पवत्परिकीर्तिता ।
सा शक्तिश्चालिता येन स मुक्तो नात्र संशयः ॥ 108

The kundalini is said to be coil shaped, like a snake. He who causes this shakti to move is liberated. Here there is no doubt.

गङ्गायमुनयोर्मध्ये बालरण्डां तपस्विनीम् ।
बलात्कारेण गृह्णीयात्तद्विष्णोः परमं पदम् ॥ 109

Forcibly grip the pitiful young widow who is between the Ganga and the Yamuna. This leads to the highest seat of Vishnu.

इडा भगवती गङ्गा पिङ्गला यमुना नदी ।
इडापिङ्गलयोर्मध्ये बालरण्डा च कुण्डली ॥ 110

The goddess Ganga is Ida. The Yamuna river is Pingala. The young widow between Ida and Pingala is kundalini.

पुच्छे प्रगृह्य भुजगीं सुप्तामुद्बोधयेच्च ताम् ।
निद्रां विहाय सा शक्तिरूर्ध्वमुत्तिष्ठते हठात् ॥ 111

Grip her tail and wake the sleeping serpent. The shakti
stirs and surges upwards.

अवस्थिता चैव फणावती सा प्रातश्च सायं प्रहरार्धमात्रम् ।
प्रपूर्य सूर्यात्परिधानयुक्त्या प्रगृह्य नित्यं परिचालनीया ॥ 112

Inhale through the sun. Grip using paridhana.[26] Make
the still serpent below move every day for an hour and a
half, morning and evening.

ऊर्ध्वं वितस्तिमात्रं तु विस्तारं चतुरङ्गुलम् ।
मृदुलं धवलं प्रोक्तं वेष्टिताम्बरलक्षणम् ॥ 113

The kanda is said to be twelve fingers above the anus, four
fingers wide, soft, white, and like a folded cloth.

सति वज्रासने पादौ कराभ्यां धारयेद्दृढम् ।
गुल्फदेशसमीपे च कन्दं तत्र प्रपीडयेत् ॥ 114

Hold the feet firmly near the ankles with the hands while
in Vajrasana and press the kanda.

वज्रासने स्थितो योगी चालयित्वा च कुण्डलीम् ।
कुर्यादनन्तरं भस्त्रां कुण्डलीमाशु बोधयेत् ॥ 115

---

[26] A secret process to be learned from a guru. Possibly the same as Nauli.

After making the kundalini move, the yogi should stay in Vajrasana and immediately do Bhastrika to quickly awaken the kundalini.

भानोराकुञ्चनं कुर्यात्कुण्डलीं चालयेत्ततः ।
मृत्युवक्त्रगतस्यापि तस्य मृत्युभयं कुतः ॥ 116

Contract the sun,[27] then make the kundalini move. Where is the fear of death even for one inside the mouth of death?

मुहूर्तद्वयपर्यन्तं निर्भयं चालनादसौ ।
ऊर्ध्वमाकृष्यते किंचित्सुषुम्नायां समुन्नता ॥ 117

Draw kundalini up a little inside the Sushumna by fearlessly making her move for as long as ninety-six minutes.

तेन कुण्डलिनी तस्याः सुषुम्नाया मुखं ध्रुवम् ।
जहाति तस्मात्प्राणोऽयं सुषुम्नां व्रजति स्वतः ॥ 118

The kundalini surely leaves the mouth of the Sushumna by doing this. Then the prana enters the Sushumna on its own.

तस्मात्संचालयेन्नित्यं सुखसुप्तामरुन्धतीम् ।
तस्याः संचालनेनैव योगी रोगैः प्रमुच्यते ॥ 119

---

[27] Located near the navel.

So make the comfortably sleeping kundalini move every day. The yogi is rid of diseases just by making her move.

येन संचालिता शक्तिः स योगी सिद्धिभाजनम् ।
किमत्र बहुनोक्तेन कालं जयति लीलया ॥ 120

The yogi who makes the shakti move is a receptacle of powers. Why say more here? He playfully conquers death.

ब्रह्मचर्यरतस्यैव नित्यं हितमिताशिनः ।
मण्डलाद्दृश्यते सिद्धिः कुण्डल्यभ्यासयोगिनः ॥ 121

Only one who delights in brahmacharya, always eats a suitable, moderate diet, and engages in the practice of kundalini will see success after forty days.

कुण्डलीं चालयित्वा तु भस्त्रां कुर्याद्विशेषतः ।
एवमभ्यसतो नित्यं यमिनो यमभीः कुतः ॥ 122

In particular, do Bhastrika after making the kundalini move. Where is the fear of death for the yogi who practices like this every day?

द्वासप्ततिसहस्राणां नाडीनां मलशोधने ।
कुतः प्रक्षालनोपायः कुण्डल्यभ्यसनादृते ॥ 123

What else but the practice of kundalini can wash away the impurities of the seventy-two thousand nadis?

इयं तु मध्यमा नाडी दृढाभ्यासेन योगिनाम् ।
आसनप्राणसंयाममुद्राभिः सरला भवेत् ॥ 124

The middle nadi of yogis is straightened by the steady practice of asanas, pranayama, and mudras.

अभ्यासे तु विनिद्राणां मनो धृत्वा समाधिना ।
रुद्राणी वा परा मुद्रा भद्रां सिद्धिं प्रयच्छति ॥ 125

Rudrani[28] (or another mudra) gives good results to those who practice energetically and hold the mind with samadhi.

राजयोगं विना पृथ्वी राजयोगं विना निशा ।
राजयोगं विना मुद्रा विचित्रापि न शोभते ॥ 126

Asanas are not useful without Raja Yoga. Kumbhaka is not useful without Raja Yoga. Even various mudras are not useful without Raja Yoga.

मारुतस्य विधिं सर्वं मनोयुक्तं समभ्यसेत् ।
इतरत्र न कर्तव्या मनोवृत्तिर्मनीषिणा ॥ 127

Practice all breathing procedures with a concentrated mind. The wise man will not direct mental activity elsewhere.

इति मुद्रा दश प्रोक्ता आदिनाथेन शम्भुना ।
एकैका तासु यमिनां महासिद्धिप्रदायिनी ॥ 128

---

[28] Shambhavimudra.

Thus the ten mudras were described by primordial Lord Shambhu. Every one of them gives yogis great powers.

उपदेशं हि मुद्राणां यो दत्ते सांप्रदायिकम् ।
स एव श्रीगुरुः स्वामी साक्षादीश्वर एव सः ॥ 129

He alone is Sri Guru who hands down the tradition's teachings about mudras. He alone is the master, the Lord incarnate.

तस्य वाक्यपरो भूत्वा मुद्राभ्यासे समाहितः ।
अणिमादिगुणैः सार्धं लभते कालवञ्चनम् ॥ 130

One tricks time, and obtains qualities like animan, by following his teachings and concentrating on the practice of mudras.

इति हठयोगप्रदीपिकायां तृतीयोपदेशः ॥

Thus ends the third chapter in the Hatha Yoga Pradipika.

चतुर्थोपदेशः
Chapter Four

Samadhi

नमः शिवाय गुरवे नादबिन्दुकलात्मने ।
निरञ्जनपदं याति नित्यं तत्र परायणः ॥ 1

Salutations to Shiva, the guru, whose nature is nada,[1] bindu,[2] and kala.[3] One ever devoted to him goes to the unstained place.[4]

अथेदानीं प्रवक्ष्यामि समाधिक्रममुत्तमम् ।
मृत्युघ्नं च सुखोपायं ब्रह्मानन्दकरं परम् ॥ 2

Now I will reveal the proper method of samadhi. It is the destroyer of death, the means to happiness, and the best giver of the bliss of Brahman.

राजयोगः समाधिश्च उन्मनी च मनोन्मनी ।
अमरत्वं लयस्तत्त्वं शून्याशून्यं परं पदम् ॥ 3

---

[1] The inner sound, represented by the crescent beneath the dot in ॐ.
[2] The inaudible sound, represented by the dot in ॐ.
[3] Part of nada.
[4] Brahman without maya.

अमनस्कं तथाद्वैतं निरालम्बं निरञ्जनम् ।
जीवन्मुक्तिश्च सहजा तुर्या चेत्येकवाचकाः ॥ ४

Raja Yoga, samadhi, unmani, manonmani, amaratva, laya, tattva, shunyashunya, paramapada, amanaska, advaita, niralamba, niranjana, jivanmukti, sahaja, and turya are synonyms.

सलिले सैन्धवं यद्वत्साम्यं भजति योगतः ।
तथात्ममनसोरैक्यं समाधिरभिधीयते ॥ ५

As salt and water become one when mixed, so the unity of self and mind is called samadhi.

यदा संक्षीयते प्राणो मानसं च प्रलीयते ।
तदा समरसत्वं च समाधिरभिधीयते ॥ ६

This state of unity—when the prana decreases and the mind dissolves—is called samadhi.[5]

तत्समं च द्वयोरैक्यं जीवात्मपरमात्मनोः ।
प्रनष्टसर्वसंकल्पः समाधिः सोऽभिधीयते ॥ ७

The similar state—the identity of jivatman and paramatman, in which all thoughts disappear—is called samadhi.[6]

---

[5] Samprajnata samadhi.
[6] Asamprajnata samadhi.

राजयोगस्य माहात्म्यं को वा जानाति तत्त्वतः ।
ज्ञानं मुक्तिः स्थितिः सिद्धिर्गुरुवाक्येन लभ्यते ॥ 8

Who truly knows the greatness of Raja Yoga? Knowledge, liberation, stability, and success are obtained from the teachings of a guru.

दुर्लभो विषयत्यागो दुर्लभं तत्त्वदर्शनम् ।
दुर्लभा सहजावस्था सद्गुरोः करुणां विना ॥ 9

Renunciation of the objects of the senses, seeing of Reality, and samadhi are difficult to obtain without the compassion of a true guru.

विविधैरासनैः कुम्भैर्विविचित्रैः करणैरपि ।
प्रबुद्धायां महाशक्तौ प्राणः शून्ये प्रलीयते ॥ 10

The prana is dissolved in the Sushumna when the shakti is awakened by various asanas, kumbhakas, and mudras.

उत्पन्नशक्तिबोधस्य त्यक्तनिःशेषकर्मणः ।
योगिनः सहजावस्था स्वयमेव प्रजायते ॥ 11

Samadhi appears automatically in the yogi whose shakti is awake and who has abandoned all actions.

सुषुम्नावाहिनि प्राणे शून्ये विशति मानसे ।

तदा सर्वाणि कर्माणि निर्मूलयति योगवित् ॥ 12

The knower of Yoga uproots all actions when the prana flows in the Sushumna and the mind enters the void.[7]

अमराय नमस्तुभ्यं सोऽपि कालस्त्वया जितः ।
पतितं वदने यस्य जगदेतच्चराचरम् ॥ 13

Salutations immortal! You even conquered time, into whose mouth this world of moving and unmoving fell.

चित्ते समत्वमापन्ने वायौ व्रजति मध्यमे ।
तदामरोली वज्रोली सहजोली प्रजायते ॥ 14

Amaroli, Vajroli, and Sahajoli are attainable once the mind has achieved identity and the breath moves in the middle.

ज्ञानं कुतो मनसि संभवतीह तावत्
प्राणोऽपि जीवति मनो म्रियते न यावत् ।
प्राणो मनो द्वयमिदं विलयं नयेद्यो
मोक्षं स गच्छति नरो न कथंचिदन्यः ॥ 15

How can wisdom emerge in the mind as long as the prana lives and the mind does not die? Whoever leads this pair (prana and mind) to dissolution is liberated. No one else, not by any means.

---

[7] Brahman.

ज्ञात्वा सुषुम्नासद्भेदं कृत्वा वायुं च मध्यगम् ।
स्थित्वा सदैव सुस्थाने ब्रह्मरन्ध्रे निरोधयेत् ॥ 16

Always reside in a good place. Know proper opening
of the Sushumna. Make the breath go into the middle.
Restrain it in the Brahmarandhra.

सूर्याचन्द्रमसौ धत्तः कालं रात्रिंदिवात्मकम् ।
भोक्त्री सुषुम्ना कालस्य गुह्यमेतदुदाहृतम् ॥ 17

Sun and moon give time the form of day and night.
Sushumna is the eater of time. This is declared to
be a secret.

द्वासप्ततिसहस्राणि नाडीद्वाराणि पञ्जरे ।
सुषुम्ना शाम्भवी शक्तिः शेषास्त्वेव निरर्थकाः ॥ 18

There are seventy-two thousand nadi passages in the
body. Sushumna is the Shiva power. The remainder have
no purpose.

वायुः परिचितो यस्मादग्निना सह कुण्डलीम् ।
बोधयित्वा सुषुम्नायां प्रविशेदनिरोधतः ॥ 19

The practiced breath enters the Sushumna without
restriction after awakening the kundalini and the
gastric fire.

सुषुम्नावाहिनि प्राणे सिद्धद्यत्येव मनोन्मनी ।
अन्यथा त्वितराभ्यासाः प्रयासायैव योगिनाम् ॥ 20

Manonmani is definitely attained when the prana flows in
the Sushumna. If it weren't, practices for the other nadis
would be mere drudgery for the yogis.

पवनो बध्यते येन मनस्तेनैव बध्यते ।
मनश्च बध्यते येन पवनस्तेन बध्यते ॥ 21

He who binds the breath, binds the mind. He who binds
the mind, binds the breath.

हेतुद्वयं तु चित्तस्य वासना च समीरणः ।
तयोर्विनष्ट एकस्मिंस्तौ द्वावपि विनश्यतः ॥ 22

The two causes of the mind are vasanas and breath.
When one perishes, both perish.

मनो यत्र विलीयेत पवनस्तत्र लीयते ।
पवनो लीयते यत्र मनस्तत्र विलीयते ॥ 23

The breath dissolves where the mind dissolves. The mind
dissolves where the breath dissolves.

दुग्धाम्बुवत्संमिलितावुभौ तौ तुल्यक्रियौ मानसमारुतौ हि ।
यतो मरुत्तत्र मनःप्रवृत्तिर्यतो मनस्तत्र मरुत्प्रवृत्तिः ॥ 24

Like milk and water blended together, mind and breath have the same action. Where there is breath, there is thinking. Where there is mind, there is breathing.

तत्रैकनाशादपरस्य नाश एकप्रवृत्तेरपरप्रवृत्तिः ।
अध्वस्तयोश्चेन्द्रियवर्गवृत्तिः प्रध्वस्तयोर्मोक्षपदस्य सिद्धिः ॥ 25

When one is active, the other is active. When one perishes, the other perishes. If these two don't perish, the group of senses is active. If these two perish, the state of liberation is attained.

रसस्य मनसश्चैव चञ्चलत्वं स्वभावतः ।
रसो बद्धो मनो बद्धं किं न सिद्ध्यति भूतले ॥ 26

Mercury and the mind are naturally unsteady. What on earth is unattainable when mercury and mind are bound?

मूर्च्छितो हरते व्याधीन्मृतो जीवयति स्वयम् ।
बद्धः खेचरतां धत्ते रसो वायुश्च पार्वति ॥ 27

O Parvati! When steady, mercury and the breath carry away diseases. When dead, they give life. When bound, they enable one to move in the sky.

मनःस्थैर्ये स्थिरो वायुस्ततो बिन्दुः स्थिरो भवेत् ।
बिन्दुस्थैर्यात्सदा सत्त्वं पिण्डस्थैर्यं प्रजायते ॥ 28

When the mind is firm, the breath is firm, then the
semen is firm. Strength and a firm body always result
from firm semen.

इन्द्रियाणां मनो नाथो मनोनाथस्तु मारुतः ।
मारुतस्य लयो नाथः स लयो नादमाश्रितः ॥ 29

The mind is the lord of the senses, but the breath is the
lord of the mind. Laya is the lord of the breath, and that
laya depends on nada.

सोऽयमेवास्तु मोक्षाख्यो मास्तु वापि मतान्तरे ।
मनःप्राणलये कश्चिदानन्दः संप्रवर्तते ॥ 30

This may be called liberation, or in another's opinion, it
may not be. Nonetheless, indescribable bliss ensues when
there is laya of mind and prana.

प्रनष्टश्वासनिश्वासः प्रध्वस्तविषयग्रहः ।
निश्चेष्टो निर्विकारश्च लयो जयति योगिनाम् ॥ 31

The laya of the yogis—inhalation and exhalation ceased,
grasping of objects destroyed, inactive, unchanging—
is supreme.

उच्छिन्नसर्वसंकल्पो निःशेषाशेषचेष्टितः ।
स्वावगम्यो लयः कोऽपि जायते वागगोचरः ॥ 32

When all thoughts are destroyed and all actions eliminated, laya is born, known by oneself, beyond the realm
of words.

यत्र दृष्टिर्लयस्तत्र भूतेन्द्रियसनातनी ।
सा शक्तिर्जीवभूतानां द्वे अलक्ष्ये लयं गते ॥ ३३

Where there is sight, there is laya. Ignorance (which always
exists in the senses and the elements) and the shakti of
living beings attain laya in the one without characteristics.

लयो लय इति प्राहुः कीदृशं लयलक्षणम् ।
अपुनर्वासनोत्थानालयो विषयविस्मृतिः ॥ ३४

They say, "laya laya." What is the nature of laya? Laya is
forgetting objects because vasanas don't recur.

वेदशास्त्रपुराणानि सामान्यगणिका इव ।
एकैव शाम्भवी मुद्रा गुप्ता कुलवधूरिव ॥ ३५

The Vedas, Shastras, and Puranas are like common
courtesans. Only one, Shambhavimudra, is protected like
a respectable woman.

अन्तर्लक्ष्यं बहिर्दृष्टिनिमेषोन्मेषवर्जिता ।
एषा सा शाम्भवी मुद्रा वेदशास्त्रेषु गोपिता ॥ ३६

The observable is inside; the unblinking gaze is outside.
This is the Shambhavimudra preserved in the Vedas
and Shastras.

अन्तर्लक्ष्यविलीनचित्तपवनो योगी यदा वर्तते
दृष्ट्या निश्चलतारया बहिरधः पश्यन्नपश्यन्नपि ।
मुद्रेयं खलु शाम्भवी भवति सा लब्धा प्रसादाद्गुरोः
शून्याशून्यविलक्षणं स्फुरति तत्तत्त्वं परं शाम्भवम् ॥ 37

When the yogi remains with mind and breath dissolved
in the internal object, seeing outside and below with
motionless pupils, and even then not seeing, this is indeed
Shambhavimudra. If it is obtained from the grace of a
guru, then that Reality, which is other than void or not
void and belongs to Shambhu, manifests.

श्री शाम्भव्याश्च खेचर्या अवस्थाधामभेदतः ।
भवेच्चित्तलयानन्दः शून्ये चित्सुखरूपिणि ॥ 38

Sri Shambhavi and Khechari—despite differences of
position[8] and place[9]—create in the void the bliss of the
laya of the mind, which has the form of consciousness
and happiness.

तारे ज्योतिषि संयोज्य किंचिदुन्नमयेद्भ्रुवौ ।

---

[8] Of the eyes.
[9] Focus of meditation.

पूर्वयोगं मनो युञ्जन्नुन्मनीकारकः क्षणात् ॥ ३९

Join the pupils in the light.[10] Raise the brows a little.
Concentrate the mind as in the aforesaid practice. This
will quickly make unmani.

केचिदागमजालेन केचिन्निगमसंकुलैः ।
केचित्तर्केण मुह्यन्ति नैव जानन्ति तारकम् ॥ ४०

Some are perplexed by the web of scriptures, some by the
contradictions in ritualistic works, some by logic. They
do not know the raft.[11]

अर्धोन्मीलितलोचनः स्थिरमना नासाग्रदत्तेक्षण-
श्चन्द्रार्कावपि लीनतामुपनयन्निस्पन्दभावेन यः ।
ज्योतीरूपमशेषबीजमखिलं देदीप्यमानं परं
तत्त्वं तत्पदमेति वस्तु परमं वाच्यं किमत्राधिकम् ॥ ४१

Eyes half closed, mind steady, sight given to the tip of
the nose, dissolving even moon and sun with the state of
immobility, one goes to the highest object, the goal, the
seed of everything, the highest Reality, which is blazing,
all encompassing, and has the form of light. What more
can be said here?

दिवा न पूजयेल्लिङ्गं रात्रौ चैव न पूजयेत् ।

---

[10] Seen when concentrating on the tip of the nose.
[11] Unmani, on which one crosses the ocean of Samsara.

सर्वदा पूजयेल्लिङ्गं दिवारात्रिनिरोधतः ॥ 42

Do not worship the Atman by day. Do not worship the
Atman at night. Always worship the Atman by halting
day and night.

सव्यदक्षिणनाडिस्थो मध्ये चरति मारुतः ।
तिष्ठते खेचरी मुद्रा तस्मिन्स्थाने न संशयः ॥ 43

The breath, staying in the left and right nadis, goes
into the middle. The Khecharimudra lives in that place,
without a doubt.

इडापिङ्गलयोर्मध्ये शून्यं चैवानिलं ग्रसेत् ।
तिष्ठते खेचरी मुद्रा तत्र सत्यं पुनः पुनः ॥ 44

The void in the middle of Ida and Pingala swallows the
breath. There stands Khecharimudra. This is definitely
the truth.

सूर्यचन्द्रमसोर्मध्ये निरालम्बान्तरं पुनः ।
संस्थिता व्योमचक्रे या सा मुद्रा नाम खेचरी ॥ 45

In the middle of sun and moon, in the unsupported space
in the circle of the void,[12] there lies the mudra known
as Khechari.

---

[12] Between the brows.

सोमाद्यत्रोदिता धारा साक्षात्सा शिववल्लभा ।
पूरयेदतुलां दिव्यां सुषुम्नां पश्चिमे मुखे ॥ 46

It is truly Shiva's beloved. Cover the unequaled, divine
Sushumna at the back opening[13] where the stream flows
from the moon.

पुरस्ताच्चैव पूर्येत निश्चिता खेचरी भवेत् ।
अभ्यस्ता खेचरी मुद्राप्युन्मनी संप्रजायते ॥ 47

Fill it[14] at the front[15] also. That is definitely Khechari.
When practiced, Khecharimudra itself becomes unmani.

भ्रुवोर्मध्ये शिवस्थानं मनस्तत्र विलीयते ।
ज्ञातव्यं तत्पदं तुर्यं तत्र कालो न विद्यते ॥ 48

Shiva's place is between the brows. There the mind
dissolves. That state is known as turya. There, time is not.

अभ्यसेत्खेचरीं तावद्यावत्स्याद्योगनिद्रितः ।
संप्राप्तयोगनिद्रस्य कालो नास्ति कदाचन ॥ 49

Practice Khechari until the Yoga sleep arrives. Time
never exists for one in the Yoga sleep.

---

[13] With the tongue.
[14] With prana.
[15] Bottom opening.

निरालम्बं मनः कृत्वा न किंचिदपि चिन्तयेत् ।
स बाह्याभ्यन्तरे व्योम्नि घटवत्तिष्ठति ध्रुवम् ॥ 50

Make the mind supportless. Don't think of anything.
Be just like a pot—space outside and inside.

बाह्यवायुर्यथा लीनस्तथा मध्यो न संशयः ।
स्वस्थाने स्थिरतामेति पवनो मनसा सह ॥ 51

As the external breath is dissolved, so is the internal,
without a doubt. The breath, with the mind, attains
stillness in its own place.[16]

एवमभ्यस्यतस्तस्य वायुमार्गे दिवानिशम् ।
अभ्यासाज्जीयते वायुर्मनस्तत्रैव लीयते ॥ 52

The breath of one practicing this way day and night in the
path of breath is dissolved. Then the mind also dissolves.

अमृतैः प्लावयेद्देहमापादतलमस्तकम् ।
सिद्ध्यत्येव महाकायो महाबलपराक्रमः ॥ 53

Drench the body with nectar from the head to the soles
of the feet. One will definitely get a great body, and great
strength and heroism.

---

[16] Sushumna.

शक्तिमध्ये मनः कृत्वा शक्तिं मानसमध्यगाम् ।
मनसा मन आलोक्य धारयेत्परमं पदम् ॥ 54

Center the mind in the shakti and the shakti in the mind.
Observe the mind with the mind, then concentrate on
the highest state.

खमध्ये कुरु चात्मानमात्ममध्ये च खं कुरु ।
सर्वं च खमयं कृत्वा न किंचिदपि चिन्तयेत् ॥ 55

Center the self in space and space in the self. Make everything space, then don't think of anything.

अन्तः शून्यो बहिः शून्यः शून्यः कुम्भ इवाम्बरे ।
अन्तः पूर्णो बहिः पूर्णः पूर्णः कुम्भ इवार्णवे ॥ 56

Empty within, empty without, empty like a pot in space.
Full within, full without, full like a pot in the ocean.

बाह्यचिन्ता न कर्तव्या तथैवान्तरचिन्तनम् ।
सर्वचिन्तां परित्यज्य न किंचिदपि चिन्तयेत् ॥ 57

Don't think of external things and don't think of internal
things. Abandon all thoughts, then don't think of anything.

संकल्पमात्रकलनैव जगत्समग्रं
संकल्पमात्रकलनैव मनोविलासः ।

संकल्पमात्रमतिमुत्सृज निर्विकल्प-
माश्रित्य निश्चयमवाप्नुहि राम शान्तिम् ॥ 58

The entire universe is just a creation of thought. The play of the mind is just a creation of thought. Abandon the mind which is only thought. Take refuge in the changeless, O Rama, and surely find peace.

कर्पूरमनले यद्द्वत्सैन्धवं सलिले यथा ।
तथा संधीयमानं च मनस्तत्त्वे विलीयते ॥ 59

As camphor in fire, like salt in water, so the mind immersed in Reality dissolves.

ज्ञेयं सर्वं प्रतीतं च ज्ञानं च मन उच्यते ।
ज्ञानं ज्ञेयं समं नष्टं नान्यः पन्था द्वितीयकः ॥ 60

The knowable, the known, and knowledge—all are said to be the mind. When knowledge and the knowable are lost, there is no second path.[17]

मनोदृश्यमिदं सर्वं यत्किंचित्सचराचरम् ।
मनसो ह्युन्मनीभावाद्द्वैतं नैवोपलभ्यते ॥ 61

All this, whether mobile or immobile, is a presentation of the mind. Duality is not obtained from the mind's state of unmani.

---

[17] No duality.

ज्ञेयवस्तुपरित्यागाद्विलयं याति मानसम् ।
मनसो विलये जाते कैवल्यमवशिष्यते ॥ 62

The mind dissolves from abandoning knowable things.
After the mind is dissolved, kaivalya remains.

एवं नानाविधोपायाः सम्यक्स्वानुभवान्विताः ।
समाधिमार्गाः कथिताः पूर्वाचार्यैर्महात्मभिः ॥ 63

Thus are the paths to samadhi, consisting of various sorts
of methods told by the great, ancient teachers following
their own correct experience.

सुषुम्नायै कुण्डलिन्यै सुधायै चन्द्रजन्मने ।
मनोन्मन्यै नमस्तुभ्यं महाशक्त्यै चिदात्मने ॥ 64

Salutations to you, Sushumna, kundalini, nectar born
of the moon, manonmani, great power in the form
of consciousness.

अशक्यतत्त्वबोधानां मूढानामपि संमतम् ।
प्रोक्तं गोरक्षनाथेन नादोपासनमुच्यते ॥ 65

The cultivation of nada—taught by Gorakshanatha,
suitable even for the ignorant who are incapable of
knowing Reality—is now treated.

श्री आदिनाथेन सपादकोटिलयप्रकाराः कथिता जयन्ति ।
नादानुसंधानकमेकमेव मन्यामहे मुख्यतमं लयानाम् ॥ 66

One and one-quarter crores of methods of laya told by
Shiva still flourish. We think only one, concentration on
nada, is the most important of the layas.

मुक्तासने स्थितो योगी मुद्रां संधाय शाम्भवीम् ।
शृणुयाद्दक्षिणे कर्णे नादमन्तस्थमेकधीः ॥ 67

The yogi, staying in Muktasana and holding the Shambhavimudra, should listen single-mindedly to the sound
within the right ear.

श्रवणपुटनयनयुगलघ्राणमुखानां निरोधनं कार्यम् ।
शुद्धसुषुम्नासरणौ स्फुटममलः श्रूयते नादः ॥ 68

Close the holes of the ears, both eyes, the nose, and
the mouth. A clear, clean sound is heard in the pure
Sushumna channel.

आरम्भश्च घटश्चैव तथा परिचयोऽपि च ।
निष्पत्तिः सर्वयोगेषु स्यादवस्थाचतुष्टयम् ॥ 69

There are four stages in all Yogas: arambha, ghata,
parichaya, and nishpatti.

ब्रह्मग्रन्थेर्भवेद्भेदो ह्यानन्दः शून्यसंभवः ।
विचित्रः क्वणको देहेऽनाहतः श्रूयते ध्वनिः ॥ 70

When the knot of Brahman is split, the sound not struck—causing bliss, arising in the void, polyphonic, tinkling—is heard in the body.

दिव्यदेहश्च तेजस्वी दिव्यगन्धस्त्वरोगवान् ।
संपूर्णहृदयः शून्य आरम्भो योगवान्भवेत् ॥ 71

When the sound in the void[18] begins, the practitioner of Yoga will have a divine body, radiance, a divine fragrance, freedom from disease, and a full heart.

द्वितीयायां घटीकृत्य वायुर्भवति मध्यगः ।
दृढासनो भवेद्योगी ज्ञानी देवसमस्तदा ॥ 72

In the second stage, the breath unites[19] and enters the middle.[20] The yogi will then be firm in asanas, wise, and an equal of the gods.

विष्णुग्रन्थेस्ततो भेदात्परमानन्दसूचकः ।
अतिशून्ये विमर्दश्च भेरीशब्दस्तदा भवेत् ॥ 73

---

[18] Anahata chakra.
[19] With apana, nada, and bindu.
[20] The middle chakra, Vishuddhi.

Then there is a pounding kettledrum sound in the extreme void[21] indicative of the highest bliss from splitting the knot of Vishnu.

तृतीयायां तु विज्ञेयो विहायोमर्दलध्वनिः ।
महाशून्यं तदा याति सर्वसिद्धिसमाश्रयम् ॥ 74

In the third stage, the sound of a drum in space is discerned. Then the breath enters the great void,[22] the repository of all powers.

चित्तानन्दं तदा जित्वा सहजानन्दसंभवः ।
दोषदुःखजराव्याधिक्षुधानिद्राविवर्जितः ॥ 75

After the bliss of the mind is transcended, the bliss of the natural state appears. The yogi will be free of defects, misery, old age, disease, hunger, and sleep.

रुद्रग्रन्थिं यदा भित्त्वा शर्वपीठगतोऽनिलः ।
निष्पत्तौ वैणवः शब्दः क्वणद्वीणाक्वणो भवेत् ॥ 76

In nishpatti, the breath goes to the seat of Shiva after splitting the knot of Rudra. There is a flute sound and a vibrating vina sound.

एकीभूतं तदा चित्तं राजयोगाभिधानकम् ।

[21] Vishuddhi chakra.
[22] Ajna chakra.

सृष्टिसंहारकर्तासौ योगीश्वरसमो भवेत् ॥ 77

The unification of the mind is called Raja Yoga. That yogi, maker of creation and destruction, is equal to Ishvara.

अस्तु वा मास्तु वा मुक्तिरत्रैवाखण्डितं सुखम् ।
लयोद्भवमिदं सौख्यं राजयोगादवाप्यते ॥ 78

Let there be, or let there not be, liberation—undisturbed happiness is right here. This pleasure arising from laya is obtained from Raja Yoga.

राजयोगमजानन्तः केवलं हठकर्मिणः ।
एतानभ्यासिनो मन्ये प्रयासफलवर्जितान् ॥ 79

I consider those practitioners who only do Hatha, without knowing Raja Yoga, to be laboring fruitlessly.

उन्मन्यवाप्तये शीघ्रं भ्रूध्यानं मम संमतम् ।
राजयोगपदं प्राप्तुं सुखोपायोऽल्पचेतसाम् ।
सद्यः प्रत्ययसंधायी जायते नादजो लयः ॥ 80

In my opinion, meditating between the brows speeds the attainment of unmani. It's an easy way for those of small intellect to achieve the state of Raja Yoga. Laya born of nada quickly produces experience.

नादानुसंधानसमाधिभाजां योगीश्वराणां हृदि वर्धमानम् ।
आनन्दमेकं वचसामगम्यं जानाति तं श्रीगुरुनाथ एकः ॥ 81

Unequaled, unutterable bliss grows in the hearts of good
yogis experiencing samadhi by concentrating on nada.
Only a great guru knows it.

कर्णौ पिधाय हस्ताभ्यां यं शृणोति ध्वनिं मुनिः ।
तत्र चित्तं स्थिरीकुर्याद्यावत्स्थिरपदं व्रजेत् ॥ 82

The sage should fix his mind on that sound, which he
hears after closing his ears with his hands, until he attains
the steady state.

अभ्यस्यमानो नादोऽयं बाह्यमावृणुते ध्वनिम् ।
पक्षाद्विक्षेपमखिलं जित्वा योगी सुखी भवेत् ॥ 83

Practicing this sound masks exterior sounds. The yogi will
be happy after eliminating all distractions for a fortnight.

श्रूयते प्रथमाभ्यासे नादो नानाविधो महान् ।
ततोऽभ्यासे वर्धमाने श्रूयते सूक्ष्मसूक्ष्मकः ॥ 84

Various loud sounds are heard in the first stage of practice.
Subtler and subtler ones are heard as the practice grows.

आदौ जलधिजीमूतभेरीझर्झरसंभवाः ।

मध्ये मर्दलशङ्खोत्था घण्टाकाहलजास्तथा ॥ 85
अन्ते तु किङ्किणीवंशवीणाभ्रमरनिःस्वनाः ।
इति नानाविधा नादाः श्रूयन्ते देहमध्यगाः ॥ 86

These are the various sounds heard in the middle of the
body. In the beginning: ocean, cloud, kettledrum, and
jharjhara drum. In the middle: drum and conch, bell and
drum. In the end: tinkling bell, flute, vina, and a bee.

महति श्रूयमाणेऽपि मेघभेर्यादिके ध्वनौ ।
तत्र सूक्ष्मात्सूक्ष्मतरं नादमेव परामृशेत् ॥ 87

Concentrate only on the subtler than subtle sound, even
when loud sounds like a cloud, a kettledrum, and so
on are heard.

घनमुत्सृज्य वा सूक्ष्मे सूक्ष्ममुत्सृज्य वा घने ।
रममाणमपि क्षिप्तं मनो नान्यत्र चालयेत् ॥ 88

Don't move the unsteady mind elsewhere, even though
it's playing on a subtle thing after leaving a gross one,
or on a gross thing after leaving a subtle one.

यत्रकुत्रापि वा नादे लगति प्रथमं मनः ।
तत्रैव सुस्थिरीभूय तेन सार्धं विलीयते ॥ 89

The mind steadies immediately in whatever sound it
adheres to first, then dissolves together with the sound.

मकरन्दं पिबन्भृङ्गो गन्धं नापेक्षते यथा ।
नादासक्तं तथा चित्तं विषयान्नहि काङ्क्षते ॥ 90

As a bee drinking honey ignores the fragrance, so the mind dissolved in nada surely doesn't desire objects.

मनोमत्तगजेन्द्रस्य विषयोद्यानचारिणः ।
समर्थोऽयं नियमने निनादनिशिताङ्कुशः ॥ 91

This sharp stick of nada can control the mind roaming in the garden of objects like a noble elephant in rut.

बद्धं तु नादबन्धेन मनः संत्यक्तचापलम् ।
प्रयाति सुतरां स्थैर्यं छिन्नपक्षः खगो यथा ॥ 92

The mind—bound by the chain of nada, its unsteadiness gone—becomes completely still, like a bird whose wings are clipped.

सर्वचिन्तां परित्यज्य सावधानेन चेतसा ।
नाद एवानुसंधेयो योगसाम्राज्यमिच्छता ॥ 93

One who desires the kingdom of Yoga should abandon all mental activity and, with an attentive mind, concentrate on nada alone.

नादोऽन्तरङ्गसारङ्गबन्धने वागुरायते ।

अन्तरङ्गकुरङ्गस्य वधे व्याधायतेऽपि च ॥ 94

Nada is like a net that catches the deer of the mind. It's also like a hunter who kills the deer of the mind.

अन्तरङ्गस्य यमिनो वाजिनः परिधायते ।
नादोपास्तिरतो नित्यमवधार्या हि योगिना ॥ 95

Concentration on nada corrals the horse of the yogi's mind. Therefore the yogi should attend to it every day.

बद्धं विमुक्तचाञ्चल्यं नादगन्धकजारणात् ।
मनः पारदमाप्नोति निरालम्बाख्यखेऽटनम् ॥ 96

The mercury of the mind is bound by mixing it with the sulfur of nada. Unsteadiness gone, it moves in the sky called Brahman.

नादश्रवणतः क्षिप्रमन्तरङ्गभुजङ्गमः ।
विस्मृत्य सर्वमेकाग्रः कुत्रचिन्नहि धावति ॥ 97

Upon hearing nada, the snake of the mind quickly forgets everything, becomes absorbed, and doesn't slither anywhere.

काष्ठे प्रवर्तितो वह्निः काष्ठेन सह शाम्यति ।
नादे प्रवर्तितं चित्तं नादेन सह लीयते ॥ 98

Fire burning in wood ceases with the wood. The mind turned towards nada dissolves with the nada.

घण्टादिनादसक्तस्तब्धान्तःकरणहरिणस्य ।
प्रहरणमपि सुकरं शरसंधानप्रवीणश्चेत् ॥ 99

Even hitting the deer of the mind is easy if it's motionless, riveted by the sound of a bell, etc., and one is skilled in the aiming of arrows.[23]

अनाहतस्य शब्दस्य ध्वनिर्य उपलभ्यते ।
ध्वनेरन्तर्गतं ज्ञेयं ज्ञेयस्यान्तर्गतं मनः ।
मनस्तत्र लयं याति तद्विष्णोः परमं पदम् ॥ 100

The knowable exists inside the audible reverberation of the sound not struck. The mind unites with the knowable and dissolves there. It is the highest seat of Vishnu.

तावदाकाशसंकल्पो यावच्छब्दः प्रवर्तते ।
निःशब्दं तत्परं ब्रह्म परमात्मेति गीयते ॥ 101

The idea of space exists as long as there is sound. The soundless is said to be the highest Brahman and the highest Atman.

यत्किंचिन्नादरूपेण श्रूयते शक्तिरेव सा ।

---

[23] In the control of prana.

यस्तत्त्वान्तो निराकारः स एव परमेश्वरः ॥ 102

Whatever is heard in the form of nada is definitely shakti. The formless, who is the end of the elements, is indeed the highest Lord.

सर्वे हठलयोपाया राजयोगस्य सिद्धये ।
राजयोगसमारूढः पुरुषः कालवञ्चकः ॥ 103

All the methods of Hatha and laya are for achieving Raja Yoga. The man who has scaled Raja Yoga is a deceiver of time.

तत्त्वं बीजं हठः क्षेत्रमौदासीन्यं जलं त्रिभिः ।
उन्मनी कल्पलतिका सद्य एव प्रवर्तते ॥ 104

Mind is the seed, Hatha the field, indifference the water. Unmani, the desire-granting creeper, sprouts immediately with these three.

सदा नादानुसंधानात्क्षीयन्ते पापसंचयाः ।
निरञ्जने विलीयेते निश्चितं चित्तमारुतौ ॥ 105

Accumulated sins are eliminated by always concentrating on nada. Mind and breath definitely dissolve in the unstained.

शङ्खदुन्दुभिनादं च न शृणोति कदाचन ।

काष्ठवज्जायते देह उन्मन्यावस्थया ध्रुवम् ॥ 106

With the state of unmani, one surely never hears the sound of a conch or dundubhi drum, and the body becomes wooden.

सर्वावस्थाविनिर्मुक्तः सर्वचिन्ताविवर्जितः ।
मृतवत्तिष्ठते योगी स मुक्तो नात्र संशयः ॥ 107

The yogi who is completely released from all states and free of all thoughts remains as if dead. He is liberated. Here there is no doubt.

खाद्यते न च कालेन बाध्यते न च कर्मणा ।
साध्यते न स केनापि योगी युक्तः समाधिना ॥ 108

The yogi in samadhi is neither eaten by time, nor bound by Karma, nor overpowered by anyone.

न गन्धं न रसं रूपं न च स्पर्शं न निःस्वनम् ।
नात्मानं न परं वेत्ति योगी युक्तः समाधिना ॥ 109

The yogi in samadhi knows neither smell, nor taste, nor form, nor touch, nor sound, nor himself, nor others.

चित्तं न सुप्तं नो जाग्रत्स्मृतिविस्मृतिवर्जितम् ।
न चास्तमेति नोदेति यस्यासौ मुक्त एव सः ॥ 110

One whose mind is neither asleep nor awake, free of remembering and forgetting, doesn't perish or flourish. That one is indeed liberated.

न विजानाति शीतोष्णं न दुःखं न सुखं तथा ।
न मानं नापमानं च योगी युक्तः समाधिना ॥ 111

The yogi in samadhi knows neither heat nor cold, misery nor happiness, honor nor dishonor.

स्वस्थो जाग्रदवस्थायां सुप्तवद्योऽवतिष्ठते ।
निःश्वासोच्छ्वासहीनश्च निश्चितं मुक्त एव सः ॥ 112

Healthy, apparently sleeping while in the waking state, without inhalation and exhalation—only he is unequivocally liberated.

अवध्यः सर्वशस्त्राणामशक्यः सर्वदेहिनाम् ।
अग्राह्यो मन्त्रयन्त्राणां योगी युक्तः समाधिना ॥ 113

The yogi in samadhi is invulnerable to all weapons, beyond the power of all people, and beyond the grip of mantras and yantras.

यावन्नैव प्रविशति चरन्मारुतो मध्यमार्गे
यावद्विन्दुर्न भवति दृढः प्राणवातप्रबन्धात् ।
यावद्ध्याने सहजसदृशं जायते नैव तत्त्वं

तावज्ज्ञानं वदति तदिदं दम्भमिथ्याप्रलापः ॥ 114

As long as the moving breath doesn't enter the Sushumna,
as long as the semen is not firmed by breath control, and
as long as the meditating mind is unlike the natural state,
talk of true knowledge is arrogant, deceitful chatter.

इति हठयोगप्रदीपिकायां चतुर्थोपदेशः ॥

Thus ends the fourth chapter in the Hatha Yoga Pradipika.

Contributors

BRIAN DANA AKERS began practicing Hatha Yoga at age twelve, learning Sanskrit at seventeen, and working in publishing at twenty-three. You can find out more about him at BrianDanaAkers.com.

ॐ

JILL ALERA BUTSON, the woman in the photographs, loves sharing Yoga with other people. She also works full-time caring for ill, injured, and orphaned wildlife.
MICHAEL L. RIXSON has been a professional photographer since 1983 and a practitioner of Yoga since 1997.

ॐ

YOGAVIDYA.COM is dedicated to publishing excellent and affordable books about Yoga. It is completely independent of any commercial, governmental, educational, or religious institutions.